THE
INNER
RACE

PURSUING YOUR POTENTIAL AT
THE CROSSROADS OF MIDLIFE

NATALIA LAZARUS

Cover and interior formatting by KUHN Design Group | kuhndesigngroup.com

The Inner Race: Pursuing Your Potential at the Crossroads of Midlife
First published by Lazarus Wellness 2025
Copyright © 2025 by Natalia Lazarus

ISBN Paperback: 979-8-9898070-5-5
ISBN eBook: 979-8-9898070-6-2

For more information, visit www.NataliaLazarus.com

I dedicate this book to my loving parents and grandparents,
who nurtured my running journey from a young age.

To my husband, soulmate, and best friend, Ryan,
who has run alongside me metaphorically and
physically throughout this incredible journey of life.

To my teenagers, Cienna and Easton, who challenge me
to show up as the best version of myself. You inspire me
to stay curious about life and keep going when it's hard.

And to all of you who dare to dream—
it's yours to chase. Go for it!

CONTENTS

FOREWORD

When I first met Natalia, what struck me immediately was her vibrant energy, an unmistakable, enlivened spark that radiated in her presence. She wasn't just chasing a big dream; she was answering something much deeper, a call that came from inside her, clear and undeniable.

We met the day before she dreamed up the title *The Inner Race*, and even in those early conversations, there was no mistaking the fire she carried. She wasn't just inspired by the idea of running The Great World Race; she was moved by it, lit up from the inside out. There was a deep recognition between us, two women standing at the edge of possibility, willing to trust what was calling them forward. What stayed with me most wasn't just her ambition; it was her wonder, that tender, electric space where everything felt possible.

I had the privilege of walking alongside Natalia during the season when this book was born. As her creative embodiment coach, I watched her not only run, but unravel, remember, and rise. Each chapter felt like a mile marker in Natalia's return to her essence. I witnessed her reclaim her voice, not just as a runner, coach, or mother, but as a woman willing to run the long road inward.

Opening a book like this is no small act. It signals a kind of readiness, a willingness to pause, to question, and perhaps, to meet yourself anew. It is an act of quiet bravery to even pick up a book that whispers there is more for you. It asks something rare: your openness, your heart, and your willingness to imagine a new way forward. In a world obsessed with outer milestones, this book chooses a more courageous path, the path inward. *The Inner Race* isn't about chasing bigger goals for the sake of achievement. It is about remembering the inner spark you carry and daring to let it catch fire again.

Natalia invites you to set an inspired movement challenge, not to prove anything, but to remember everything you already are. Her story reminds us that the real race isn't measured in miles, but in how fully we come alive. Reading these pages, I found myself reflecting on the creative process I know so intimately, how initial sparks of inspiration eventually give way to doubt, fatigue, and the uncomfortable necessity of trust. Watching Natalia navigate the writing of this book mirrored the very journey she describes, the one where momentum fades, and what remains is devotion, an unwavering trust that the dream was given to you for a reason, and that the dream is meant to be pursued.

If you are holding this book, you may be standing at your own threshold. May Natalia's words remind you that you do not need to know exactly where you are going, only that you are willing to take the first step. And the next.

You are already in motion.
The race has already begun.
Trust the pull within you, and find your inner race.

KELLY WILDE MILLER, CREATIVE EMBODIMENT COACH

1

IGNITE YOUR SPARK

"Your vision will become clear only when you look into your own heart. Who looks outside, dreams; who looks inside, awakens."

CARL JUNG

t was winter a few years back when something in me began to stir. For the first time in years, I found myself pausing long enough to take a breath. My daughter was getting ready for high school, my son was officially a teenager, and just like that, the stage of being the overscheduled, overextended mom of little kids was over. I had navigated the sleepless nights, the early morning chaos of packing lunches and finding lost shoes, the after-school shuttling between soccer practice and baseball games, all while managing conference calls, deadlines, and the invisible mental load of keeping a household running.

I had spent years running on autopilot, moving from one task to the next, constantly needed, constantly responsible. And then, suddenly, the house was quieter. The kids no longer needed me in the same way. No one was clinging to my leg or calling for me in the middle of the night. I wasn't buried in birthday party invitations or PTA emails. For the first time in a long time, I had space to breathe.

And with that breath came gratitude, deep, overwhelming gratitude. For the years spent rocking babies to sleep, for the early morning walks to school while they held my hand, for the laughter echoing from the backseat during long drives. Every beautiful moment has shaped me, filled my heart, and given my life meaning in ways I could never have imagined. I'd do it all over again in a heartbeat.

But as the chaos settled, a new, unfamiliar question emerged: Now what?

For so long, my identity had been woven into being a mother, a wife, a professional, a caretaker, the glue that held everything together. My purpose had been crystal clear: nurture, support, and create a life where my family could thrive. But as my children grew more independent, I felt something unexpected creeping in, not relief, but a quiet emptiness. Who was I when I wasn't constantly rushing, planning, or managing someone else's schedule?

For years, I had poured everything into my family, often putting myself last. And now, with this new space in my life, I realized I wasn't even sure what I wanted anymore.

I tried filling the space with more work, more house projects, more trips and travel adventures, and yes, more scrolling on my phone, but none of it satisfied the restlessness I felt deep inside. I had checked all the boxes of what I was "supposed" to do: build a career, raise healthy, happy kids, and keep the house running, but I couldn't shake the feeling that somewhere along the way, I had lost myself. That fire

I once had, the passion, the ambition, the energy all felt like a distant memory.

I wasn't burned out; I just felt disconnected from the version of me that had once dreamed, pushed herself, and chased goals just for the thrill of it.

I needed something to wake me up, to reignite the spark I had lost. But where did I even begin?

As these thoughts swirled in my mind, growing louder by the day, my family and I arrived in Newport Beach for a weekend away. That's when I did something I hadn't done in a long time. I set out on my own, left my family to relax at the hotel, laced up my running shoes, and went for a run on the beach.

My legs felt heavy, my breath was labored, and my stride was out of sync in a way it hadn't been before. But I kept going. Running along the coastline on an unfamiliar trail, I found myself not just exploring new terrain but also navigating the uncharted territory of my own thoughts.

That run shook off the dust. It was the moment that brought me the clarity I had been searching for.

In a culture where most of us weren't given the tools to navigate the potentially unsettling transition of midlife, I found myself searching for a way to reconnect with my inner spark.

I had to actually listen to the roommate in my head I had been ignoring for so long.

My path, and the one I feel compelled to share with you in this book, was to set a challenge that would inspire me to grow and evolve into this next phase of life. A challenge focused on movement. Why movement? Because when movement and inner work align, the impact isn't just incremental—it's exponential.

Let's pause for a moment: What exactly is movement?

While broad terms like fitness and workout often carry connotations of struggle, discipline, or the pursuit of weight loss, movement is something deeper; it's an expression of our physical bodies, a way to connect with ourselves on a fundamental level. Unlike rigid exercise routines that can feel like an obligation, movement is fluid, adaptable, and personal. It's not just about burning calories or achieving a certain aesthetic; it's about feeling alive, strong, and in sync with your body.

Movement comes in many forms: walking, yoga, playing, recreation, sports, strength training, dancing, cycling, hiking, swimming, and, yes, running! It can be structured or spontaneous, high-energy or restorative, solo or social. The key is to find movement that excites and fulfills you, something that not only strengthens your body but also creates space for self-reflection, clarity, and growth. When you approach movement as a tool for transformation rather than a chore, it becomes a powerful catalyst for both physical and inner change.

REIGNITE

We all share the human experience of transitioning to different life stages, stages where the direction is clear and your inner spark is a raging fire, and stages where we feel a bit lost or disconnected and the spark is barely a pilot light. If you are currently in the latter stage, like I was, I promise the light is still on, and there is beauty and power in seeing this stage for what it is. If you're ready to connect with your inner spark, the power of setting an inspired movement challenge can ignite your potential and passion.

Like so many women in midlife, I felt disoriented by the sudden shift from constantly caring for others to suddenly having more space. Society celebrates young adulthood and achievement-driven milestones, but what happens when the demands quiet down? The transition can bring an unsettling mix of emotions, including relief, loss, freedom, and uncertainty.

Without the structure of past roles, I felt disconnected from my former self, grappling with a loss of purpose and fearing that the best years were behind me. This identity shift, often unrecognized or unsupported by societal norms, can trigger an internal crisis, one where external accomplishment no longer defines a clear path forward.

But what if this phase isn't an ending but an invitation to rediscover who you truly are?

What if, instead of feeling lost, this transition became the moment you reconnect with your passions, redefine your purpose, and step into the most empowered version of yourself?

I knew I needed something to reignite my inner spark. That's when I turned back to running, my lifelong compass. Running has always given me clarity, a place to process life's transitions, and a way to reconnect with myself. This time, it wasn't just about fitness; it was about pursuing a movement challenge to find *me* again. To truly understand how deeply running had shaped my life and identity and to rediscover the spark it once ignited, I had to return to where it all began.

A RUNNER'S JOURNEY

As a child, carefree and focused on playing with friends and siblings, running was fun and usually part of a game of tag or hide and seek. It didn't require any thought, effort or equipment and was always part of a larger expression of childhood.

In elementary school, the first time I connected with running on a deeper level was in PE with my first-ever mentor, Miss Dalton. She was one of those rare teachers who left a lasting impact, and she was the first person to challenge me to run fast.

As the oldest of four siblings, I suppose I was always competing in some way, seeking attention within a busy family, but I had never really competed against my peers. That changed in Miss Dalton's 7th-grade PE class when she announced we'd be participating in the Presidential Physical Fitness Test. If we met all the required metrics, including a timed one-mile run, we would earn an award.

The challenge immediately excited me. It was as if all I needed was a goal, a time to chase, and I could pour all my energy into achieving it. I should mention that most of my classmates found the test silly and annoying, putting in little effort. But I took it seriously; it sparked something in me. And while that spark has, at times, faded to little more than a pilot light, in those early years, it was a fire.

I ran that mile as if it were an Olympic race, outrunning all my peers except for the two fastest boys in school. I was hooked.

From that point on, I would run anywhere I could. Why walk home from school when I could run? It made me feel alive, strong, and confident and connected me with a part of myself that was new and exciting. This stage of my life was pure love of running, no expectations, just exploration.

A few days before starting high school at Justin-Siena, a small private school in the Napa Valley, I was still carrying with me this love of running when I learned about all the sports the school offered. That was the first time I heard about cross-country. I vividly remember coming home and excitedly telling my parents, "Guess what? There is a high school sport called cross-country, where all you do is run!"

Up until that point, I had only associated running with other sports like soccer or basketball, where being a strong runner was important but never the main goal. I had never excelled in those traditional team sports; I played them just to be with my friends and have fun. But discovering that I could focus on and compete in the one thing I knew I could do well felt like a dream come true.

That freshman-year team was special. We connected easily across all grade levels, boys and girls, JV and Varsity, different backgrounds and interests. We'd meet up in the parking lot with our super sweet but very old coach, Coach D. We'd chat, lace up our shoes, and he'd give us a route to run for the day. I'm not sure we ever really warmed up, stretched, or had any conversations about proper running mechanics, injury prevention, or nutrition. We just ran.

In a way, that was a gift. There were no expectations and no pressure to perform. Cross-country had always been an overlooked part of our high school athletics department, but in my freshman year, we changed that.

When I started racing, I felt that fire within me; I wanted to push my personal limits as far as I could. I began treating practices like races, sometimes competing only against myself. Beat my last PR. Beat the course record. Learn to embrace the pain cave, that inevitable moment in a race when exhaustion sets in, your legs feel like lead, and your mind begs you to stop.

Our home cross-country course was a dusty, hilly trail system with no shade, and we ran it during the peak of Northern California's heat. On this course, passing someone meant pushing through the relentless sun, maintaining speed uphill, and taking your chances on the uneven downhill terrain. The final quarter mile demanded an all-out sprint, where only those willing to drain every last ounce of energy, push past burning lungs and aching legs and embrace the discomfort could make their move.

That season was a mental training ground for me as much as a physical one, one I look back on with gratitude as a pivotal and transformative point in my life.

Like great teams do, we all got better together. We went to the State Championships that year and proudly ran our hearts out for ourselves, our team and our school. I came back with a new and fully formed identity as a 15-year-old; I was now a "runner."

This identity of being a runner, so clear and focused in those early years, would shift as life moved through different stages. And with each change, the same question would surface:

"Am I still a runner?

In college at Santa Clara University, I walked onto the crew team. I missed being part of an organized sport and a team. More than that, I missed the structure and hard work that came with being a student-athlete. Rowing gave me all of that, along with 4 a.m. wake-up calls in 45-degree weather, frozen knuckles, and cleaning boats before my 8 a.m. classes.

But by the end of that season, I realized that for me, it wasn't just any sport that filled that void; it was running.

In my sophomore year, I walked onto the cross-country team, hoping to reconnect with the version of myself who had thrived and led my high school team with confidence. I trained all summer with the team before the season started, running more miles and at a faster pace than ever before. Most of the girls had been recruited and were already in their second or third season. I admired them, but I quickly realized I was no longer the leader; I was barely keeping up.

After months of intense training and overtraining, without fully understanding the importance of nutrition and recovery, I ended up with a double stress fracture, one in each leg, on my left and right medial tibia. I was out for the season after running just one race, and I spent the next few months in a boot and hobbling around campus on crutches.

"So, if I'm not racing in cross-country, am I still a runner?" I found myself asking again.

During the rest of my college experience, running just became fun again. I'd run for me, to clear my mind before a big exam and to connect with friends. I'd still find ways to push myself into that pain cave, just to make sure I could still handle it, but it wasn't in a structured team format anymore. It was on my terms, my time, and back in the pure love of running phase from my childhood.

What I've always loved about running is its simplicity. All you need is a pair of shoes, and the journey begins. It can be fast or slow, short or long, alone or with friends. You can think in silence or listen to music, follow a planned route, or simply explore. It can be in the dark or light, in heat or cold, on pavement or trails, none of which changes the essence of the run itself. Whatever you're seeking on any given day, running offers it. That's why it has always been my compass: constant, reliable, and adaptable to whatever I need in the moment.

In my senior year of college, I met my now husband, Ryan. One of our first dates was a run together; well, it was more like a race to see who was faster. Over the years, we have both had our moments of winning, and I think that has been a great mirror of our relationship, challenging and cheering each other on, always alongside one another for the journey.

After college, I returned to the same magical high school cross-country team in Napa, California, this time as an assistant coach and mentor. I could no longer keep up with the team the way I used to, but I ran alongside them in training and cheered them on during races.

At the same time, I signed up for my first marathon, the San Diego Rock 'n' Roll Marathon. I figured I'd give distance running a try since my faster days were behind me. While I'd love to say that I was instantly hooked, that 26.2 miles felt like my calling, and that it all came easily, it didn't. I overtrained, under-fueled, and crossed the finish line injured, exhausted, and ready to take a long break from running.

"If I'm not a cross-country runner, not a marathon runner, am I still a runner?" I wondered.

REIGNITING YOUR INNER SPARK

Every journey has its compass, that one thing that has always guided you back to yourself, no matter how far you've drifted. For me, it has always been running, but running is not for everyone. Maybe it's the feeling of strength you once found in the weight room, the achievement of summiting a mountain, the freedom of an early morning swim, the rhythm of cycling down an open road, or the quiet presence of yoga on your mat.

But what if movement has never been your compass?

Maybe your sense of purpose has always come from achievement, creativity, caregiving, or connection. Perhaps you've found fulfillment in creative endeavors like art or music, building a career, raising a family, or pursuing passions that had nothing to do with physical challenge. And yet, as life shifts, when careers plateau, bodies change, children grow, or the things that once defined you start to feel less certain, it's easy to feel unsure of what's next.

This is where movement becomes more than just exercise. It becomes a way to reconnect with yourself. Unlike external goals, movement is something you create, experience, and feel within. It challenges you, builds resilience, and shifts your perspective, not just physically but mentally, emotionally, and even spiritually.

You don't have to be a runner, a cyclist, or an elite athlete. Movement can be as simple as walking in nature, stretching on your yoga mat, or dancing to music that moves your soul. It's not about competition; it's about awakening something inside of you that has been dormant for too long.

This is your invitation to reconnect. Reconnect to anything that interests or inspires you. To step back into the space that once made you feel confident, free, and fully yourself. To rediscover the passion, the clarity—the inner fire that has been there all along.

The Inner Race is the transformative practice of setting an inspiring movement challenge, and it's what I'll be teaching in the following chapters. If you are navigating this middle stage of life, and you are looking to reconnect to your inner spark through an inspired movement challenge, this book can be your guide. We'll explore ways to reconnect and rediscover what fuels your inner fire, helping you move from feeling stuck to finding inspiration.

• • •

Pause & Reflect: What has been your guiding compass during life's transitions? Is there a recurring activity or passion from childhood that brought you joy?

Coaching Advice: Life moves in seasons; some stages call for pushing forward, while others require slowing down. Reflect on the stage you're in now. Are you in a season of challenge, recovery, or growth? Identify one activity that consistently brings you clarity and purpose.

Start Small: Journal about what brings you joy or a sense of accomplishment. Commit to one action per week that aligns with your passions, like walking, meditating, or exploring a new hobby.

Next, we'll look at how to redefine yourself in midlife and reconnect with your goals and passions.

2

REDEFINE MIDLIFE

"Be not afraid of going slowly,
be afraid only of standing still."

CHINESE PROVERB

s this it? Have I accomplished everything I thought I would by this age? Is there more?

The question starts as a whisper, then grows louder. Have you known someone who suddenly splurged on an expensive car or extravagant trips, hoping to recapture a lost spark? Or someone who became obsessed with reversing time, diving into extreme dieting or cosmetic procedures in an attempt to look young again? Maybe you've seen a friend or colleague abruptly walk away from a career or abandon responsibilities without a clear plan, more restless than truly inspired. Others seek validation through reckless romantic choices or affairs, convinced that something new will make them feel alive again. These responses, though common, are often just distractions from the real issue: a longing for purpose, identity, or a deep knowing that they have more to offer.

Have you ever felt this way yourself?

MIDLIFE ~~CRISIS~~ METAMORPHOSIS

We are all familiar with the term "Midlife Crisis." A period of self-reflection and emotional turmoil in middle age triggered by a desire to reassess life choices, achievements, and purpose. You may have experienced this first-hand or know someone who has made a drastic life change in the face of this transition. It's a feeling of being lost or uncertain that can stir up fear and lead to emotionally charged decisions. Yet, it doesn't have to remain that way; in fact, recognizing it can open up a world of opportunity.

I believe that we can shift our feelings about this cultural phenomenon and reframe it as an opportunity to move from crisis to metamorphosis.

I've spent a lot of time reflecting on why the midlife "crisis" has become such a cultural norm. The transition from raising young, dependent children to parenting more independently is a profound life shift, yet often lacks the acknowledgment or structure of a formal "rite of passage" in our culture. While we ceremonially celebrate stages like graduation, marriage, childbirth, and retirement, this particular stage is largely unmarked and thus easily can become a very lonely and isolated solo adventure. It was for me.

Parents who have spent a decade or two centering their lives around raising children are often left with a loss of purpose and identity. It's our goal to raise kids who become independent and prepared to "leave the nest," but there is a sense of loss that is a huge part of this process. The absence of a clear milestone can make it difficult to recognize this phase as an opportunity rather than a crisis.

But midlife is not an ending; it's an open invitation to redefine yourself, set new challenges, and step into the most authentic version of who you are becoming.

If you're experiencing this phase, or know someone who is, know that you are not alone. I believe it's a normal, necessary, transformative part of life's extraordinary journey.

The 40-year mark was a milestone for me, and I felt a deep need to create my own rite of passage and honor this new season in life. If you haven't heard this term before, a "rite of passage" is a ceremonial or symbolic event marking a significant transition in a person's life, often signifying personal growth and transformation. It doesn't have to be a party or a celebration in a traditional way; it can be anything that is authentic to you and your personal transformation.

Celebrating this significant birthday felt deeply important. As if I needed to pause and reflect on the decades behind me and honor who I had become. It took months to find a way to celebrate that felt true to me. I'll share the full story in an upcoming chapter, but here's a hint: it involved running.

YOU'VE DONE THIS BEFORE

Middle age may feel like uncharted territory, but it's not the first big transition you've navigated. You've adapted before, moving from childhood to young adulthood, stepping into careers, relationships, and possibly parenthood. Each phase of life has required you to evolve, to let go of what was, and to step into something new. This stage is no different. The uncertainty you may feel now is simply another invitation to grow, to redefine yourself, and to embrace what comes next with the same resilience and courage that has carried you this far. Consider this well-known parable that explains the paradox of life stages we all encounter.

"In youth, you have time and energy but no *money*.

In adulthood, you have money and energy but no *time*.

In old age, you have time and money but no *energy*."

Perhaps you've been fortunate enough to experience all three at once, and I wholeheartedly wish that for everyone. This very relatable paradox reminds us that there is a constant shift of resources—time, energy, and money—in each stage of life. It's the balance of these resources and the understanding of where you are in your life stage that will help you tap into what you need and share what you've learned along the way.

LIFE STAGE CHANGES

In the early stages of life, transitions tend to come quickly and easily; you're eager, excited, and ready for the next phase. Whether it's school, friendships, sports, new experiences, or new challenges, you move from one milestone to the next with a sense of curiosity and momentum. However, as you enter midlife or parenthood, things start to change. This stage is still filled with excitement and hustle, but it can also feel overwhelming as new responsibilities and shifts in priorities emerge.

Within each stage of life, there are transitions that force growth and evolution. Moments that challenge you to rethink who you are and what you want from life. Though these shifts can be uncomfortable and may stir fears of losing the identity you've known or how others know you, they ultimately lead to deeper understanding and lasting transformation.

Walking alongside my friend Jess during a very challenging time in her life helped me to really start connecting the dots about the power of movement to support us in rediscovering our spark. She shares her journey about how running became a catalyst for navigating a major life change.

RUNNING THROUGH GRIEF: JESS'S STORY

When my mom died, I felt like I was drowning. I knew it was coming; Alzheimer's had been taking her mind piece by piece for years, but when she was actually gone, it hit me in a way I wasn't prepared for. I had spent so much time taking care of her, managing doctors' appointments and medications, and just sitting with her, holding her hand while she slipped further away. And then, one day, there was nothing left to do. I felt lost.

At first, I just went through the motions. I barely slept and barely ate. I avoided friends because I didn't know how to answer their questions when they asked how I was doing. The house was quiet and full of sadness.

One morning, while digging through my closet, I found my old running shoes. I don't even remember what I was looking for and don't know what made me pull them out. I hadn't run in years, and I wasn't in the mood to start that day. But a sudden sense of curiosity hit me, so I put them on anyway and stepped outside. I had to get out of the house.

I told myself I'd just walk around the block. I had no plan, no goal. But somewhere along the way, my walk turned into a slow jog. My body was clunky and uncomfortable; my knees were achy, and my lungs felt like they might explode. But for the first time in weeks, I felt something other than sadness.

The next day, that sense of curiosity competed with that emotion of sadness, so I went out again. And the day after that. Some days, I barely made it a mile. Other days, I ran farther than I thought I could. I cried a lot while I ran. Sometimes, I talked to my mom in my head. Other times, I just focused on the sound of my feet hitting the pavement. It didn't take the pain away, but it gave me a way to move through it.

After a few months, that curiosity rolled into a sense of inspiration, and I signed up for a 10K in my mom's honor. Not because I was trying to prove anything, but because running had become my way back, a tool to channel my sadness. When I crossed the finish line, I wasn't just finishing a race—I was finally stepping into life again.

I've learned that grief doesn't go away, and you can't outrun it. But you can move with it. You can keep going, even when it hurts. And for me, running is how I learned to do that.

REDEFINE

Let's pause for a moment to check in and reflect on what chapter of life you are in right now. Think about what your role once was and how it has shifted. What tasks and responsibilities defined your daily life in the past? Maybe it was changing diapers, preparing meals, and running errands for your kids or elderly parents. Now, take a moment to reflect on how your days look now. What has changed? As your role as a parent or caregiver evolves, your career interests shift, or you simply find yourself in a season of life that no longer feels the same. This new chapter is the perfect opportunity to redefine your identity.

Your daily routine and priorities may have shifted, so it's beneficial to recognize these changes and take a moment to process any feelings or emotions that arise before proceeding.

Once you're ready, this phase can be an opportunity to reassess your goals, reignite your passions, and carve out space for your own aspirations. This shift is empowering; it's time to focus on what you want next and reclaim ownership of your life and dreams.

RECONNECT

This phase also gives you a chance to reconnect with yourself in ways you might have neglected during the busy years of intensive parenting, caregiving, or career-building.

Consider this moment an opportunity for personal growth. Consider it an invitation to rediscover your passions. You might want to explore enrolling in a class, starting a new project, or revisiting a creative activity that once sparked joy and fulfillment. Embrace this chance to reconnect with what inspires you.

Use this time as a chance to pour into yourself, fostering your own growth and tapping into potential that may have been dormant for years.

REFRAME

Shifting your identity during this phase can feel like a deep, unsettling process. For me, it was a scary and emotional transition. I found myself stuck, overwhelmed by the fear of change and the uncertainty of what may lie ahead. It forced me to go inward, to search for tools and practices I had never considered before. It was, at times, an uncomfortable process, but eventually, I was able to surrender and embrace it with gratitude.

I'm not alone in feeling this way; many people experience similar shifts during midlife. There's often societal pressure to have everything figured out and to have accomplished certain milestones in order to feel worthy of moving into the next phase of life. But I've learned that it's not about meeting others' expectations; it's about embracing your own evolution and letting go of what no longer serves you.

Change, while uncomfortable, is a necessary part of growth. And when you face it head-on, you'll find yourself emerging stronger, more aligned, and ready for the next chapter of your life.

MIDLIFE IS NOT AN ENDING—
IT'S AN INVITATION.

It's a time to move forward with intention, to reconnect with the passions that once inspired you, to explore the parts of life you may have set aside, and to embrace the possibilities that still await you. If you're holding this book, curious about reigniting your inner spark through an inspiring movement challenge, get excited! Movement is more than just exercise; it's a powerful metaphor for momentum, transformation, and self-discovery.

When physical movement aligns with inner growth, that's when the magic happens.

. . .

Pause & Reflect: Which "season" of life are you currently in? How does it shape your priorities, energy, and time? What is your favorite way to incorporate movement into your day?

Coaching Advice: Take out a sheet of paper and create three columns labeled *Past, Present,* and *Future.*

- *Past:* List all the ways you enjoyed moving earlier in life, including playful activities from childhood.

- *Present:* Write down your current movement habits.

- *Future:* List movements you'd like to try, perhaps something new or something you haven't done in years.

This reflection helps you recognize patterns, rediscover past joys, and set intentions for the future.

Pick one movement from your list that excites you. In the next chapter, we'll explore how movement shapes self-perception.

3

MOVE WITH PURPOSE

*"Movement is a medicine for creating change in
a person's physical, emotional, and mental states."*

CAROL WELCH

I've coached hundreds of individuals through physical transformations, but the most profound shifts don't just happen in the body; they happen in the mind. When movement is simply about burning calories or checking a workout off the list, progress is slow, uninspired, and often unsustainable. However, when movement becomes a tool for inner growth, and every run, lift, or stretch is infused with intention, the results are exponential.

Strength training becomes a practice in resilience, running teaches endurance in the face of life's challenges, yoga cultivates flexibility in both body and mindset, and play is all about having fun. I've seen it firsthand: the clients who pair movement with a deeper inner goal don't just improve; they evolve. They break through limiting beliefs, develop unshakable confidence, and build momentum that carries over into every aspect of their lives. This is the real secret to transformation; it's not just about what you do but who you become in the process.

As both an athlete and a coach, I first noticed this pattern in myself. I would get excited to try a new sport or sign up for a race, and the process of learning and training would spark transformation in other areas of my life. As I paid closer attention, I saw the same powerful shift occur in the athletes I coached in the gym; it was undeniable. Today, I share this approach with all my clients, and I'll be sharing it with you throughout these pages.

Pairing a movement goal or practice with an inner challenge creates a powerful synergy that amplifies both physical and inner transformation.

This concept is rooted in the idea that movement is not just about physical fitness but also serves as a vehicle for personal growth, self-discovery, and mindset shifts. When these two elements align, the benefits become astronomical because they reinforce and accelerate each other.

WHY THIS WORKS:

Embodied Learning: When you tie an inner challenge (e.g., overcoming self-doubt, building resilience, processing change, or developing discipline) to a movement-based challenge, your body reinforces the mental and emotional shifts. The act of physically pushing through discomfort mirrors the mental process of breaking through limiting beliefs. For example, strength-based training can be very intimidating to a beginner, but it can also be a path to overcoming self-doubt.

One of my favorite parts of coaching is empowering new athletes and teaching them to first acknowledge that by showing up to class, they've already done the hardest part. Just showing up is the first step to overcoming self-doubt. Each class offers more confidence, the movements become more familiar, and the heavy weights start to feel lighter. They are building strength in both their bodies and their minds. In just a few weeks, everyone can see their enthusiasm and confidence when they show up in class; it's a remarkable change.

Feel Good Chemistry: When you move, you feel good! Movement increases the release of "Hope Molecules," dopamine, serotonin, endorphins, hormones and other neurotransmitters that enhance mood, motivation, and clarity. This biochemical shift reinforces the work you are putting in and makes it easier to stay committed to both the physical and inner challenges.

Have you ever heard of the runner's high? It's not specific to running. It's the magical effect of all these chemicals released, coupled with a feeling of accomplishment. These chemicals provide a sense of creativity, clarity, and confidence. Don't believe me? Try it for yourself.

Rewiring Your Identity: Think back to the first time you rode a bike or skied down the mountain; how did you feel? The combination of a physical challenge (like running a marathon, lifting heavier weights, or mastering a yoga pose) with an inner challenge (such as improving self-confidence or embracing discipline) rewires your self-perception.

Every time you show up for your physical practice, you reinforce the belief that you are capable, strong, and committed to growth.

I experienced this myself when I began my yoga journey late in life. With decades spent running fast and lifting heavy, I knew deep down I was missing a restorative practice. I knew I needed to incorporate some form of flexibility and mobility. In fact, there are three pillars of movement that everyone should integrate into their routine.

1. Cardiovascular Pulmonary Endurance

2. Strength, Power, and Resistance

3. Flexibility, Mobility, and Stability

I realized I was missing the third pillar, and I was curious about yoga, so I decided to give it a shot. My first few yoga classes were a struggle. I was confused by the movements and the teacher's commands, which everyone else seemed to understand. It felt like I was in a dance class, and everyone else knew the dance moves but me. But I was committed to showing up for this practice, and eventually, I became familiar with the flow, which made me feel confident both on the mat and throughout the rest of my day.

Physical Struggle Reflects Inner Growth: When your body experiences discomfort and adapts, your mind does the same. Facing physical challenges teaches patience, grit, and resilience, traits that directly apply to your mental and emotional pursuits.

While the phrase "no pain, no gain" is extreme, the foundation of the phrase has some validity. I believe a better term may be **"No Challenge, No Change!"**

If you only train your muscles to the point of slight discomfort and quit when it becomes hard, your muscles will not have the opportunity to adapt and rebuild even stronger. When you push past the point of discomfort (holding a plank or a wall sit until your muscles start to shake), you not only build back those muscles stronger, but the sense of achievement you feel teaches you that you are capable of more than you think you are.

Momentum Effect: Momentum is a progressive, forward movement or energy in a person's life. It symbolizes the build-up of positive energy, progress, or growth because of consistent effort, focus, and dedication to health or personal goals.

This concept is often used to describe the feeling of being in a state of flow where everything seems to be moving forward harmoniously, and obstacles are overcome with ease. Progress in one area of life creates momentum in others. If you commit to a movement challenge that demands consistency, you naturally develop habits that extend beyond fitness and into relationships, career, and self-discipline in other areas.

Momentum, in this sense, represents the cumulative effect of one's efforts toward achieving a goal, manifesting as a palpable sense of progress and forward motion. It's the energy that propels us toward our aspirations, fueled by consistency, focus, and dedication.

I'm willing to bet that you've been there before. Maybe you've started waking up earlier to move your body each morning, and before you knew it, you were eating better, feeling more confident at work, being more productive around the house, and showing up with greater patience for your kids. You might have found yourself thinking more clearly, making better decisions, and feeling more in control of your day. That single commitment to consistent movement sparked a ripple effect, momentum, that carried into every corner of your life.

That's the power of progress: one aligned action unlocks another, and soon, your entire life starts moving in the direction of growth.

REAL-LIFE APPLICATIONS: MOVEMENT AND MANTRAS

Let's explore a few examples of this in real-life situations.

Pair Strength Training with Building Inner Strength

- Movement: If you struggle with self-doubt, grab a set of challenging weights.
- Mantra: With every rep, I grow stronger in body and mind.

Use Running as a Metaphor for Pushing Through Life's Challenges

- Movement: If you're navigating a tough life transition, use endurance training to reinforce persistence.
- Mantra: When I push through discomfort on my run, I remember discomfort in life is temporary, and I can keep moving forward.

Connect Yoga or Mobility Work to Flexibility in Life

- Movement: If you're working on becoming more adaptable

and open-minded, your yoga or mobility routine can be an embodied reminder to be flexible.

- Mantra: With each pose, I practice letting go, staying present, and embracing change.

Tie Cold Exposure to Mental Toughness

- Movement: If your goal is to build resilience and discipline, committing to cold plunges or ice baths helps train your nervous system to handle stress and discomfort.

- Mantra: Even when I'm deeply uncomfortable, I can sit with control and surrender.

COLD MORNINGS, STRONGER MIND: RILEY'S STORY

In just three minutes a day, I've taught myself to push beyond discomfort to override the instinct to run, hide, or escape. Instead of resisting, I surrender. And in surrendering, I overcome.

Beginning my morning ritual with three minutes in cold water is deeply uncomfortable, yet it kick-starts my day with a sense of achievement that nothing else can match.

I'm a mom. My life is a constant balancing act, and most days, I feel like I'm always reacting, always playing catch-up. The stress is relentless, the exhaustion real. But I refuse to let it define me. I need to prove to myself that I can do hard things, not just for me, but for them.

I take a deep breath and step in.

The cold hits me like a shockwave. My body seizes, and I fight the urge to gasp for air. I have to consciously slow my breath. Although every inch of me begs me to get out, I stay and breathe.

I grip the edge of the tub, squeezing my eyes shut. This is the moment where I either fight against the discomfort or accept it.

Eventually, the panic fades. My body doesn't warm up, but my mind does. The water is still freezing, but I no longer feel the need to escape. I stay steady and still. Three minutes, that's my goal.

When I step out, my skin is tingling, and my heart is pounding, but something inside me has shifted. The woman who hesitated at the edge is not the same as the one standing here now. I have emerged stronger, calmer, more capable. The cold is my first test of the day, and I passed with flying colors; I'm ready for whatever comes next.

GOAL VS. CHALLENGE

As you read on, you'll see the words *goal* and *challenge* used interchangeably. Are they the same? In this book, goals and challenges are not separate; they are synergistic and fuel each other.

- A goal is a specific target to work toward. It provides a reason to endure the challenges.

- A challenge is focused on mindset and resilience. It adds depth and meaning to the goal's achievement.

Often, setting a goal turns into a checklist, and when challenges arise, the goal is left unmet. However, by reframing the goal as a challenge and embracing it with a mindset of perseverance, your journey transforms. When obstacles arise, they become an opportunity for growth, turning your inspiring movement challenge into a powerful catalyst for personal transformation.

THE EXPONENTIAL BENEFITS

You don't need to lift heavy weights, push yourself to exhaustion, or do a cold plunge every day. But ideally, you're beginning to recognize the transformative power of pairing physical challenges with inner growth. The benefits are truly remarkable: enhancing mental clarity, building emotional resilience, accelerating habit formation, and driving lasting behavior change, all grounded in greater confidence and self-trust.

As you push your physical limits, you also build the capacity to handle stress and uncertainty with greater ease. The result? A higher quality of life, not just physically, but emotionally and mentally. This is more than just a fitness journey; it's a path to reclaiming your strength and potential in the next phase of life.

. . .

Pause & Reflect: Think back to a time when you accomplished a physical challenge; maybe you learned a new dance or hiked to the top of a steep trail. How did it change your perception of yourself? Write down how you felt at that moment.

Coaching Advice: Revisit your movement list from the last chapter. What was the one activity you picked? Can you think of a mantra that will align with your new movement to reinforce your personal transformation?

Start Small: Choose an inspiring movement challenge based on your past successes. For example, if hiking was on your list, is there a mountain you always wanted to summit? If so, start thinking of smaller hikes to prepare for this challenge and grab some friends to start training with you!

As you start taking action, challenges will arise. In the next chapter, we'll explore how to turn setbacks into stepping stones.

4

BEYOND THE MILES

"Run when you can, walk if you have to,
crawl if you must; just never give up."

Dean Karnazes

RUNNING INTO THE UNKNOWN:
MELISSA'S STORY

used to be someone who always played it safe. I followed the rules, made the right decisions, and stayed within the lines of what I knew. On the surface, life looked great. I had a steady career, decent health, and a routine that worked. But deep down, something felt a little off. I wasn't unhappy, but I wasn't fully alive either. It was like I was coasting, going through the motions without ever really testing my edges or reaching my potential.

Then, one evening, I met some friends for dinner, and a friend casually mentioned she had signed up for a half marathon. She wasn't a runner. She just wanted to prove to herself that she could do something hard. I laughed and said, "That sounds awful," but the idea wouldn't leave me. Long after the plates were cleared and the night was over, her words echoed in my mind. I kept thinking about our conversation all night.

A few days later, something unexpected happened. After countless internal debates and second-guessing, I did something wildly out of character: I signed up, too. No grand plan. No perfect timing. Just a quiet, instinctive decision that felt both terrifying and exhilarating. It was one of those moments that didn't seem like a big deal at the time, but looking back, it was a turning point. With one simple click, I wasn't just registering for a race; I was saying yes to discomfort, yes to growth, and yes to discovering a version of myself I had never met before.

I wasn't a runner either. I wasn't out of shape, but I also wasn't someone who just laced up shoes and ran 13.1 miles for fun. Still, something inside me wanted to find out what might happen if I tried.

That first run was brutal. My lungs burned, my feet hurt, my legs protested, and the voice in my head kept asking, "Why are you doing this?" But the next day, I went again. Then again.

The training was a challenge in every way. I had to wake up early, say no to excuses, and keep showing up even when motivation ran dry. I didn't love it at first. In fact, there were moments when I truly hated it. But slowly, something shifted. Running stopped being just about the race, and it became a mirror. It reflected back my doubt, my resilience, my strength.

Somewhere along the miles, I discovered I was actually capable of doing hard things.

I learned that being uncomfortable didn't mean I had to quit. That most of the limits I believed in were imagined. And that discipline, more than motivation, was the key to change.

When race day came, I was nervous and intimidated. But I showed up. I stood at the starting line, heart pounding, and when the gun went off, I ran. Step by step, mile by mile, I kept going. It wasn't fast or pretty, but I made it. I crossed that finish line, and something inside me cracked wide open.

Because it was never really about the race.

It was about breaking free from the version of myself that stayed small. It was about stepping into the unknown and realizing I could trust myself there.

Since then, everything has changed. I've said yes to things I used to avoid, like traveling alone, launching a side project, and speaking up when I would've stayed quiet. Running didn't just make me physically stronger; it woke me up to be a braver, fuller version of myself.

And it all started the day I stopped playing it safe and dared to challenge myself and see what else was possible.

PERSONAL GROWTH

It's completely normal to struggle with motivation, we all do from time to time. Staying motivated constantly just isn't realistic. We often look to outside sources to keep us going, but when life gets hectic or unexpected challenges pop up, it's easy to lose momentum. That's okay. The real shift happens when you start tuning into your own reasons for showing up, your personal "why," and learn to move through the discomfort instead of avoiding it.

I believe we all have an inner drive to learn and grow, and I believe it's part of what makes us human. And while this story might be about running, it's really just a placeholder for whatever challenge speaks to you. Maybe for you, it's something totally different: starting a new job, speaking your truth, learning a new skill, or navigating a difficult season of life. Whatever it is, the point is this: growth always starts when you step outside your comfort zone. That's where transformation begins.

RUNNING TO CREATE PRESENCE OF MIND

Through running, coaching, and my own path to personal growth, I've learned that success comes from daily commitment rather than waiting for the "perfect" moment to start.

Running is a metaphor for growth. Every mile represents a step forward, and depending on the mile you're in, maybe it's mile 1, or maybe it's mile 9, each mile requires a specific presence of mind because each mile comes with its own challenges and lessons.

My all-time favorite running quote is "Run the mile you're in" by Ryan Hall, an American long-distance runner and the fastest U.S. marathoner in history. He used this phrase as a personal mantra and later made it the title of his book. To me, this is a constant reminder of being fully present and not letting the past or the future take over your thoughts.

In a long race, it's easy to wish away the next 9 miles when you're in the first three and already feeling the pain in your knees, the heaviness in your legs or the blisters on your feet. It can even be dangerous to focus so far on the future, knowing you have hours of enduring the pain you are currently in before getting to the finish line. I catch myself in these thoughts on a run, and in life, and that quote helps to reset and reframe.

Where am I right now?

What can I focus on right now, so the next 9 miles don't feel daunting? How can I stay present and keep building momentum? Whether you're running a race, navigating a hectic phase of life, or facing a personal challenge, breaking it down into manageable steps is often the key to not feeling overwhelmed.

Sometimes, this comes in the form of focusing on one 5-mile increment. Sometimes, it's just making it to the next bridge or stop sign. And sometimes, I just count to ten. That's right, when you feel overwhelmed, you can break things down so small that just taking one breath or counting to ten becomes your focus. And suddenly, you're fully back in the present moment.

For me, and for many, running embodies the essence of growth: **persistence, patience, progress and presence.**

Persistence: Whatever goals you've set for yourself, it's going to require consistency, especially when motivation wanes. This means having the discipline to set your alarm to get the training in before your busy day begins and sticking with this habit day after day to build mental resilience. It also means embracing discomfort during hard runs or training days as a parallel to pushing through challenges in life. These small daily efforts will compound over time into meaningful milestones. *Persistence isn't about perfection; it's about showing up again and again, even when it's hard.*

Patience: Running and many other sports teach us that progress is gradual and not always immediately visible. Have you ever gone for your first run after taking a few months off? It's hard. It's painful. But by continuing to show up, you gradually rebuild your strength and endurance, and over time, it starts to feel easier again. With this long-term goal in mind, patience prevents burnout by encouraging sustainable progress instead of rushed results. *Patience allows you to trust the process, even when the results haven't shown up yet.*

Progress: Setbacks. Problems. Barriers. We all have them in life and in running. A bad race, an injury, or an undesired outcome can feel frustrating, but they are also opportunities to learn and adapt. These periods of recovery can be that pause needed to teach humility and connect back to the importance of listening to your body and mind. Whatever your path, each step forward, however small, builds momentum, and each misstep builds resilience. *Progress is not a straight line; it's a mix of highs, lows, and lessons that move you forward over time.*

Presence: Let's go back to the mind-body connection for a moment. On a challenging run, there's physical discomfort and mental discomfort. If the pain or discomfort in your body becomes too loud and your mind is not trained to override and push through, quitting becomes an option. Conversely, sometimes it's the mind that can talk us out of completing our training day or pushing up that hill, negotiating with itself over the thousands of reasons why not to. *Presence means tuning into your body and thoughts in real-time and choosing to stay engaged instead of checking out.*

Running offers more than just physical benefits; it literally becomes a training ground for the mind. Through persistence, you build the discipline to keep showing up. Patience teaches you to trust the process, even when progress feels slow. Every small win or setback contributes to your growth, and staying present helps you push through both physical and mental resistance. Running strengthens mental toughness, leaving you with the feeling: *"If I can run up that hill, I can handle that meeting, or have that hard conversation."* It's this resilience, cultivated mile by mile, that begins to spill over into every area of your life.

REDEFINING WHAT
A RUNNER LOOKS LIKE

If you're reading this and thinking, "This isn't for me—I'm not a runner," hang tight. I'm excited for you to read on, because you might just find pieces of yourself in these pages. I get it. I've been there too. Running can seem like it belongs to a specific group of people: the fast, the lean, the ultra-disciplined.

But here's the truth: running is for anyone who wants to run. It's not about fitting a certain image, reaching a specific mileage, or achieving a particular race time. It's about perseverance and deepening this relationship with yourself through movement. Sometimes, we all need a reminder of that, even those of us who've been running for years.

Let me share a recent moment when I had to remind myself of that very lesson.

I was sitting at a long dinner table with a group of new friends we had just met on vacation. It was so exciting getting to know everyone, and conversations bounced around the table, from funny stories about our family to meaningful reflections. There was a sense of openness in the air, that unique mix of curiosity and connection that only seems to happen when you're away from your everyday life.

The conversation shifted to my upcoming race. Naturally, the questions followed: How do you train for that? What do you eat? How do you recover? I was happy to share because I love talking about the process. But then, in the middle of it all, someone leaned back and said,

"You don't look like a runner."

I know she didn't mean anything by it. It wasn't meant to hurt. But it landed in a strange way. It caught me off guard. I smiled and shrugged it off, but inside, it stirred something I hadn't felt in a long time. That familiar voice from years ago whispered: "Do I really belong here? Am I doing this right?"

That comment clung to me longer than I expected. It poked at an old vulnerability, one I thought I'd outgrown. It made me question, just for a moment, if I still had something to prove. If being a runner meant looking a certain way, acting a certain way, or achieving something measurable on paper.

But the longer I sat with it, the clearer it became:

Running is fueled by spirit, not by image.

Here's an important lesson that I learned. Labels can box you in. They create invisible limits, just like perfectionism makes you feel like anything less than flawless isn't good enough. But running, just like life, isn't about checking all the boxes. It's about the joy of movement, the challenge of showing up for yourself, and the growth that unfolds along the way.

THE MARATHON OF LIFE

A marathon is 26.2 miles and takes the average person around four to five hours to complete. It's a long time to run, and if you sprint the first few miles, you'll likely burn out before reaching the end. A smart marathon strategy includes a balanced training plan with long runs, speed work, rest days, and recovery to prevent injury and build endurance. You pace yourself in the first half, conserve energy, and tap into your reserves for a strong finish. Throughout the race, you stay focused on hydration, fueling, and mental resilience to maintain a steady rhythm. It's the combination of persistence, smart planning, and adaptability that sets you up for success.

Just like in life, every effort you put in, every early morning, every setback, every breakthrough matters. A balanced approach allows you to sustain your energy and avoid burnout in this marathon of life. Each step forward, no matter how small, is a sign of progress and a building block toward becoming the best version of yourself. And while we all imagine that picture-perfect finish line moment, the true beauty lies in the transformation that happens along the way.

I encourage you to approach your movement challenge and other areas of life with the mindset of a marathoner. Without persistence, even the best plans can unravel. It's not just about physical stamina but about cultivating the mental and emotional endurance that sustains you. It's about developing the presence to shut out distractions and reconnect with your inner voice, where clarity and strength live.

Growth doesn't come from one heroic effort; it's the result of steady, intentional action repeated over time.

It's in those quiet, unseen miles where the real change begins. There will be moments of doubt, discomfort, and fatigue, but trust the process. Patience helps you stay grounded when results feel far away. Progress may not always be visible, but it's happening beneath the surface. And with each step, you're building something far greater than a finish line moment; you're building resilience, self-trust, and a life that reflects the strength of your journey.

• • •

Pause & Reflect: What challenge or setback have you faced recently, and what has it taught you about perseverance and growth? How can you apply those lessons moving forward?

Coaching Advice: Setbacks are learning opportunities. Instead of seeing them as failures, track them. Write down obstacles and successes, then review them regularly to identify patterns.

Start Small: Focus on consistency, not perfection; establish a routine to stay on track and create an accountability system that works for you.

Now that you've learned that obstacles are an important part of the journey, let's identify what energizes and motivates you in the next chapter.

5

REDISCOVER PASSION

"The meaning of life is to find your gift.
The purpose of life is to give it away."

PABLO PICASSO

As the years passed and my children grew older and more independent, a new reality settled in. I suddenly had more time for myself: time that used to be filled with the endless demands of motherhood. Perhaps, for those who've poured their energy into a demanding career, relationships, or other responsibilities, it's that moment when life shifts, and you're left wondering what comes next. The question that lingered for me was, "Now what?" Without the constant need to pour into others, I felt disconnected from myself and was in search of something to reignite my energy.

Then, a friend invited me to join a Saturday morning running group. At first, I hesitated because six miles before sunrise, in the cold, with women who were already strong runners felt intimidating. But I showed up anyway. Those first runs were humbling; I struggled to keep up, returning home exhausted. Yet, something about those mornings felt right. We weren't just running; we were sharing life, talking through challenges, celebrating wins, and holding each other accountable. Week after week, my body grew stronger, but more importantly, my sense of self had returned.

Running became more than just exercise again; it became a space where I could reclaim my identity, separate from the roles I had carried for so long. It reminded me that I wasn't just a mother, a professional, or a caretaker; I was still me. And I was still capable of chasing goals that were mine alone.

Many people reach a point where they've done everything they were "supposed" to: built a career, raised a family, and secured a home, yet something still feels missing. Without a clear goal or new challenge, life can start to feel limited, and doubts creep in. Is it too late to start something new? Can I really redefine my path? It's an unsettling feeling, but it's also an opportunity, and it can lead to personal growth in the journey ahead.

Of course, my journey involved running, but as I've shared, any kind of inspiring movement challenge can help you rediscover your spark. One of my clients, Ali, shares her story about how strength training helped her build physical and mental strength.

BUILDING THE STRENGTH WITHIN:
ALI'S STORY

I don't know exactly when it happened. There wasn't some big moment where I decided to stop taking care of myself. Life just got busy. Work was exhausting, my to-do list was never-ending, and honestly, I didn't feel strong enough.

But I've shown up at my strength class anyway, standing here in front of the weights, telling myself I'll just get through it. One rep at a time.

The warm-up feels sluggish. My body is stiff, my mind distracted. The voice of self-doubt sneaks in, whispering, *You're too tired. You should go easy today. You're not as strong as the others.*

I ignore it and load my bar.

The first few reps of squats are shaky, my legs are burning. But as I push through the discomfort, something shifts. My breath steadies. My stance feels stronger. The weight that seemed heavy at the start doesn't feel impossible anymore.

Halfway through the workout, my arms shake during the presses, my heart pounds from the rows. Sweat drips down my back. This is where I used to stop, where I'd let fatigue be my excuse. But today, I keep going. Every rep is a reminder: I am stronger than I think.

It's time for the final set, and instead of dread, I feel something else: determination. I can hear my coach in the background, encouraging me to keep going. I brace, lift, and finish the last round. When I rack the weights for the final time, I feel it deep in my bones.

I didn't just complete the workout; I proved something to myself.

I wipe the sweat from my face, exhausted but exhilarated. Every time I show up, I rewrite the story I've told myself for years. The one that says I'm not strong enough, not capable enough.

That story doesn't belong to me anymore.

I let this feeling soak in. I look around and see the hard work and accomplishment on the faces of everyone in the class. We'll be back tomorrow for another round.

• • •

Ali's story is a common one. It is a reminder that even if the demands of life change and taking care of ourselves moves to the bottom of the list, there is always a way to come back.

This next section comes from a place of both love and lived experience, working as a health and fitness coach and as someone who has experienced the power of setting an inspiring movement challenge in my own life. When you enter a new stage of life, setting a goal, big or small, can serve as a powerful metaphor for overcoming personal obstacles.

SET AN INSPIRED
MOVEMENT CHALLENGE

While there is always a place for setting challenges, they become especially important during life transitions or big changes because they provide a sense of direction and clarity. Before we go any deeper, just take inventory of your own personal inner fire today. Does it feel like a raging inferno ready for direction or a pilot light that needs some fuel? Wherever you are, we all have periods of life that include both ends of the spectrum and everything in between. Knowing where you are right now will help you get the most out of this next chapter.

MOTIVATION

But first, let's define a few terms. There are two types of motivation, intrinsic and extrinsic, and it's important to have a balance of both to understand your motivation behind the challenge you are setting. If the scales are tipped too far in one direction, it will become harder to reach your goal because it's out of balance.

Extrinsic goals: Extrinsic or outer goals are usually externally motivated and driven by external rewards like recognition, earning money, achieving status, or meeting others' expectations. Examples include taking on a project at work just to earn a promotion or dropping a quick 5 lbs. before the beach vacation with friends. These goals are more focused on short-term gains and can provide initial momentum, but without the balance of intrinsic motivation, they are hard to sustain.

Intrinsic goals: Intrinsic or inner goals are usually internally motivated and driven by personal values, interests, and a desire for personal growth and self-fulfillment. These goals are aligned with your sense of purpose and are pursued because they are inherently satisfying. Examples include health-driven goals like eating well so you can have more energy during the day, or mastering a new skill like creative writing, a passion of yours since childhood.

So, just like everything in life, it's a balance that creates the sweet spot of motivation in goal setting, and it's important to evaluate if your personal goal is intrinsically and/or extrinsically motivated.

Additionally, when setting goals, it's powerful to frame them in a positive, forward-moving way, focusing on what you want rather than what you're trying to avoid. For example, saying, "I want to read fiction before bed," is far more motivating than, "I want to stop doomscrolling late at night." The first gives you a clear, actionable direction, while the second keeps your mind focused on the habit you're trying to break. Sometimes, it's easy to notice what you don't want but not as easy to clearly define what you do want. Taking the time to reframe a goal in a positive way can provide clarity, making it easier to take meaningful steps forward.

Now is your chance to reframe this midlife transition as an opportunity, a time to explore and evolve. It all starts with a commitment to yourself. In just a few moments every day, you can reconnect to your inner spark and work toward an inspiring challenge.

● ● ●

Pause & Reflect: What energizes you about the movement you chose from the previous chapter? What makes you curious about it?

Coaching Advice: Reflect on the movement you've selected, and list both external (extrinsic) and internal (intrinsic) motivators. A balanced motivation source will keep you aligned and committed.

Is your motivation driven by joy, curiosity, and fulfillment, or is it based on obligation and external validation?

If your goal aligns with what excites you, you're ready to move forward!

Now, let's turn this inspiring movement goal into a concrete plan in the next chapter.

6

EMBRACE CHANGE

"It is not the mountain we conquer, but ourselves."

Sir Edmund Hillary

I didn't realize how much I needed a challenge until I committed to running 40 miles for my 40th birthday. It was a bold, seemingly impossible goal, but the training process changed me in ways I never expected.

My kids were 13 and 11 years old, excited about school, friends, and time with their cousins. My husband had a career he was passionate about and had helped so many people achieve their own health goals. My family was thriving. So why did I feel this immense pressure as this milestone birthday approached? How would I celebrate and honor my 40 years? I sat with that question for months. It just didn't feel right to celebrate with a party or a vacation. I wanted to connect with the most authentic version of myself, but I wasn't really sure what that looked like anymore.

One morning, the house was quiet. The kids were still asleep as I sat by the fire, enjoying my coffee with my golden retriever, Charlie, at my feet. Outside, the sky was beginning to lighten, and the house would come alive any minute. As I let my mind wander, an idea struck me: I decided I would run 40 miles. Not just for the challenge, but to honor every year of my life—the highs, the lows, the lessons, and the gratitude. The thought sent a surge of energy through me. I took another sip of coffee, a slow smile forming. Yeah, that's it. That's how I'll mark this milestone.

I had no idea if this was possible. Up until that moment, my longest run was a failed marathon in my twenties. But something deep inside me just knew I could and should do this. I trusted that voice, the one pushing me forward, and made a conscious decision to quiet the usual doubts and fears of failure that so often held me back. I knew deep down that failure was always a possibility, but the real power wasn't in the outcome; it was in the process of getting there.

At first, I didn't act on this dream right away. I let the idea simmer, checking in with myself to make sure it wasn't just an impulsive thought that would be forgotten in a few days. Was this goal meaningful to me beyond just proving to myself I could do it? Was it something I wanted for myself, or was I just trying to impress others? I had set goals before, that were more about external validation than personal fulfillment, and I knew the difference. But this one? This one felt different. It wasn't about finishing a certain time, earning a medal, or proving anything to anyone; it was about honoring my life journey, embracing a challenge, and seeing what I was capable of.

Once I committed, I started training: long runs with friends and solo miles during the week. My favorite moments were when my kids would wake up, hop on their bikes, and join me on the trail for the last few miles. For months, I kept the dream to myself, protecting it and letting it take shape before sharing it with anyone. When I finally told my husband, his reaction was cautious: "What if you just run 40K (25ish miles)?" I understood the skepticism; it was a big jump from anything I had ever done, but I knew in my gut that it had to be 40 miles.

With five months to train, I slowly started telling my extended family and close friends, and what began as a personal challenge quickly turned into something much bigger.

MILES AND MILESTONES

On the morning of my 40th birthday, I put on my headlamp, packed my nutrition, and, with the light of a full moon, hit the trail with Ryan. He was initially only supposed to run with me the first 10 miles but surprised me and ran a full 16 miles to celebrate the 16 years we had been married. During those miles, we ran past our first condo, where we first became parents, and remembered dreaming about what our first house would look like. We also listened to the new Stick Figure album, released the day before.

After Ryan parted ways with me, I continued the next 10 miles on my own, feeling pretty good. I even took phone calls from my mom and brother-in-law, who called to cheer me on.

Unexpectedly, while on the trail, two of my close running friends surprised me and began to run alongside me, and then another group joined in a few miles later. Suddenly, it felt like a party! Friends from all over the community joined for a few miles or more to celebrate this milestone birthday, and many ran farther than they ever had before. My daughter joined in on the fun and ran 13 miles to celebrate her upcoming 13th birthday. My son and his friends biked alongside us, while Ryan held down the meeting spot, preparing protein shakes and hydration drinks for runners coming in. Later that evening, we hosted everyone at our house to celebrate a challenge accomplished, a milestone birthday, and the love and support of family and friends.

The gratitude I feel for the support of my friends and family on that day will never be forgotten. Following your dreams can be very vulnerable and scary. This was the first time in a long time I had followed mine and pushed all those fears away. It allowed me to connect to a truer version of myself that I had not seen in a while.

Have you ever looked in the mirror and said to yourself, "There's so much more in there!" We are capable of so much, yet many of us avoid setting big challenges because of fear of failure, judgment, or self-doubt. But when we stop striving for something, or when the goal we've been working toward suddenly shifts or disappears, motivation can fade, making room for complacency to quietly settle in.

The fear of not measuring up or falling short can feel paralyzing, making it easier to stay in the comfort of routine rather than risk pursuing something uncertain. Over time, this avoidance leads to a sense of unworthiness, questioning whether it's even possible to dream big again. But the challenge is what fuels growth, and stepping outside your comfort zone, even in small ways, is the first step toward reigniting passion, purpose, and confidence.

Running has become one of my primary opportunities for inner and outer growth. Each year, I've continued to run my age, and every year, it looks a little different. Sometimes, it's a solo adventure; sometimes, I run with friends. Some years, it's hard and slow, while in others, I've trained well and felt prepared. Regardless of the circumstances, each year is a powerful reminder that, despite the changes in my running journey, it's still my way to go inward and connect to myself.

Now, when I take a break from running or have a slow day, that voice comes into my head and asks,

"Am I still a runner?"

I confidently answer,

"Yes. I am a runner. I'm also a mother, daughter, sister, wife, friend, health coach, fitness instructor, yogi, and whoever else I evolve into."

Running has been my compass, reconnecting me to who I am and who I'm becoming. I've learned that speed or distance doesn't define you—as long as you're running toward your dreams.

Connecting to this path of personal growth doesn't have to involve running at all; it can be any challenge that stretches you and inspires you! Once you commit to a goal that's balanced intrinsically and extrinsically, the next step is to set yourself up for success, making sure you accomplish smaller, more achievable goals along the way to boost your confidence and motivation for the larger goal.

COMPONENTS OF GOAL SETTING

Let's go back to the definition of challenge vs. goal. The goal is the measurable target you are chasing, and the challenge is the mindset you have as you pursue your unique movement goal.

Motivation: The brain's reward system plays a key role in keeping you motivated when pursuing a meaningful challenge. When you set a goal, anticipate success, and achieve milestones, it creates a feedback loop that reinforces effort and progress.

Self-efficacy: A core component of goal setting is your own belief in your ability to succeed. If you have high self-efficacy, you're more likely to set ambitious goals and overcome setbacks. Conversely, low efficacy can lead to avoidance of challenges and giving up before even getting started. Don't worry if your self-efficacy is low; achieving small milestones will build confidence and resilience.

Reframing: Setting a goal helps shift focus from feeling stuck to creating opportunities for self-growth. If you are struggling with a personal or professional setback, set a small goal balanced with intrinsic and extrinsic motivators and shift your energy to something you are excited about that feels achievable.

Visualization: Imagining the success of this goal can train your body and mind to believe it is achievable and helps increase focus, motivation and confidence. This can also be a fun activity where you take a moment each day and truly feel the emotions associated with accomplishing your goal. This mental rehearsal will help you make daily decisions that align with your objectives.

HOW GOALS DRIVE TRANSFORMATION

If you are in a place in life where you are transitioning from one stage to the next, such as becoming an empty nester or changing careers, setting a new goal can act as a fresh start and fill the void created by the unknown. For me, it's having teenagers who are becoming more independent, allowing me to connect to the version of myself that exists today—quite different from who I was 15 years ago before I became a mom. No matter where you are in your life right now, goals can guide you on a journey of self-discovery and help you reclaim your identity.

Setting goals also helps build resilience, which is such an important life skill. In pursuing a goal, you will inevitably learn to embrace failure as feedback, not defeat. The more this happens, the better you will become at quickly moving on to the next step in the process instead of getting stuck in the feelings of failure or defeat. This newfound mental toughness is developed through consistent effort, even when progress feels slow. You learn to refocus quickly, allowing you to get back on track.

Many people have a complicated relationship with goal setting. For some, past experiences of pushing too hard, burning out, or chasing goals that felt more like obligations than desires have left them feeling exhausted or even resistant to the idea of setting goals at all.

In this book, goal setting is not about toxic productivity, hustle culture, or the pressure to constantly achieve. Instead, we explore a healthy and intentional approach to goal setting that supports us rather than depletes us. The kind of goal setting I encourage focuses not on merely checking boxes or proving your worth through productivity, but on tapping into your inner spark and reconnecting with what truly excites you. It aims to give you a sense of direction that aligns with who you are today. When we approach goals in this way, they transform into tools for self-discovery rather than instruments of self-punishment.

Ultimately, this is an opportunity to connect with that inner joy and personal alignment that you truly deserve! A goal that you are passionate about will act as fuel for your motivation, even if things get difficult along the way. Additionally, you'll likely find that your enthusiasm for this new goal inspires those around you to make positive changes in their own lives.

GOAL SETTING 101

We've explored how goal setting can ignite your inner spark and the importance of balancing internal and external motivation. By now, you may already have an inspiring movement goal in mind. Next, let's explore your goal through the SMART goals framework, credited to George T. Doran, to help set and refine your goal.

SMART GOALS FRAMEWORK:

1. Specific: Define your goal clearly

2. Measurable: Track progress with smaller milestones

3. Achievable: Check in with yourself to make sure this goal is within reach

4. Relevant: Ensure the goal aligns with your personal values

5. Time-bound: Set a deadline to maintain focus and hold yourself accountable

The **SMART** goals framework can be used for any goal, personally or professionally. It's a great way to clearly define whatever goal you are working towards so that you set yourself up for success. As you go through the framework, if you find that you haven't set a deadline, now is your opportunity to clarify that piece of your goal. Think of it as a checks and balances approach to ensure that your investment of time and energy leads to a successful outcome.

THE FLOORS AND CEILINGS APPROACH

Goal setting isn't just about big achievements; it's about creating a realistic path to success. I like to think of goals in terms of "floors" and "ceilings," a concept commonly attributed to Brad Stulberg and Steve Magness. They introduced it in their work on performance psychology, particularly in *The Practice of Groundedness* and *Peak Performance*.

This method encourages setting a "floor" goal (the minimum, nonnegotiable effort you'll put in) and a "ceiling" goal (the ideal, best-case scenario). The idea is that having both types of goals allows for flexibility and consistency, ensuring progress even on tough days while still striving for higher achievement when possible. It's particularly effective for habit formation, training, and long-term goal success.

You don't have to sign up for a marathon to feel the power of goal setting; it's about building momentum through small, consistent wins. Many of us struggle when we set a goal so big that, after a few weeks, the energy and excitement fade, and it's easy to give up.

As a coach, I see this often in January, when clients start the year with a New Year's resolution to lose weight or start an intense fitness routine. They set a "ceiling" goal, start the year with strict rules, and hit the gym hard, but by the third week of January, they give up on their goal and slip back into old patterns. Why does this happen? Their goal was not properly supported with smaller "floor" goals to keep the momentum and motivation on days when the "ceiling" goal feels impossible or out of reach.

The real magic in goal setting is to set "floors" or smaller, more achievable goals along the way that help keep us motivated to work towards the larger "ceiling" goal we have set for ourselves.

Floors: The minimum commitment you'll make, even on tough days. These are small, realistic actions that keep you in motion so you don't lose progress.

Ceilings: The big, stretch goal you're working toward, the ideal outcome if everything goes well.

For example, if your New Year's resolution is to get back into shape by walking every day, setting both a floor and a ceiling goal can help you stay consistent without feeling overwhelmed. Your floor goal might be: "I'll take the stairs instead of the elevator," ensuring that even on busy days, you're making progress. Your ceiling goal could be: "I'll walk for one hour after work each day." This approach keeps you moving forward while allowing flexibility. By consistently hitting your floor, you build momentum and confidence, making it easier to reach your larger fitness goals over time.

• • •

Pause & Reflect: Connect back to the movement goal that inspired you. What emotions arose: excitement, hesitation, fear? Both positive and negative feelings can guide you forward.

Coaching Advice: It's time to commit to your goal and build out smaller goals to support you! Use the SMART goal framework (Specific, Measurable, Achievable, Relevant, Time-bound) and the "floors and ceilings" approach (set a minimum and maximum goal to maintain flexibility).

1. Reflect: What inspires you?

2. Find Your Why: What deeper purpose drives this goal?

3. Break It Down: Big goals (ceilings) need small, achievable steps (floors).

4. Build a Network: Who will support and uplift you?

You've now identified a movement goal that excites and challenges you, used the SMART framework to clarify your goal and supported it with smaller, more achievable "floor" goals. In the next chapter, we'll explore strategies to stay focused and block out distractions, ensuring you remain motivated and committed to achieving it.

7

ANCHOR WITHIN

*"When we are no longer able to change a situation,
we are challenged to change ourselves."*

VIKTOR E. FRANKL

NAVIGATING THE NOISE: LISA'S STORY

Lisa sat in her car outside the grocery store, staring at the steering wheel, the weight of the day pressing in from all directions. Her phone buzzed constantly: texts from her nearly grown kids about rides and last-minute plans, a voicemail from her aging mother, unread emails from work, and a reminder to finally schedule that overdue mammogram. In a fleeting attempt to escape, she opened social media and let herself get lost in the mindless scroll of other people's lives.

"When did I start feeling so disconnected," she wondered. Her days used to revolve around playdates, bedtime stories, and chasing after little kids. Now, the house was quieter, the demands were different, but the mental load was somehow heavier.

In a world filled with constant noise from social media, external expectations, and her own inner critic, it had become impossible to hear herself think, let alone feel.

If this scenario sounds familiar, you are not alone. In today's fast-paced world, there is a constant pull on our attention, from external demands like work deadlines, family obligations, and social expectations to the ever-present inner critic whispering that we should always be doing more. The noise can be deafening, making it easy to lose sight of what truly matters.

Many people struggle with feeling overwhelmed, trying to balance the expectations of busy motherhood, a demanding job, managing a household, and still finding time to get to the gym, walk the dog, and maintain a social life. The never-ending to-do list leaves little room for personal goals or inner transformation. When we pile on distractions, unhealthy habits, or toxic relationships in our workplaces or communities, it's no wonder we feel misaligned, disconnected, and exhausted. It can feel like a battlefield, with everyone demanding a piece of our time and energy until there's nothing left for ourselves. Even if the hands-on caretaking responsibilities might be lessening, there's still a constant pull on our attention.

I call this "noise."

But the path to clarity begins when we start evaluating where the "noise" is coming from and making intentional choices to eliminate what no longer serves us. When I was in my own evaluation phase, the list of distractions was long; some were easy to cut, like binge-watching my favorite shows, text threads that pinged all day, and mindless scrolling on social media. Others took much longer, like leaving a toxic workplace that drained my energy and prevented me from thriving.

It's not about making drastic changes overnight but taking one step at a time toward alignment. As you strip away distractions and reclaim your focus, you begin to uncover your values, strengths, and purpose. And in this process, you not only quiet the noise around you, but you also start to hear your true voice once more.

SYSTEM OVERLOAD

For me, profound realization wasn't something that happened overnight; it was the result of years of allowing more noise to creep into my life, not really knowing the importance of protecting my boundaries. But, as the demands of daily life continued to grow, little by little, year after year, eventually, I couldn't even hear myself think. I realized something had to change.

At the time, I had just started a new job in a stressful and unhealthy work environment, one that completely clashed with my values. Every morning felt like an uphill battle, draining me in a way I had never experienced before. This misalignment was making me miserable and depleting my energy. Some days, I felt like I had nothing left for my family, let alone myself.

I didn't know it yet, but I was on defense. I was in a reactive state, in survival mode, and my usual healthy habits and tools just weren't enough. I was struggling to keep my head above water, and I certainly wasn't thriving. It felt like I was in system overload, and something had to change—fast!

LEAN ON YOUR SUPPORT SYSTEM

If you or anyone you know have ever had to hit pause and reevaluate why things just aren't quite working in life, my hope is that you will seek out and lean on a support system. My husband, Ryan, was not only my soundboard but also the person who would lift me back up on the really tough days. He is also the creator of The Lazarus Method, a framework that eventually helped me understand which pieces of my life needed extra focus so I could rebalance and regain my health.

THE LAZARUS METHOD:
DR. RYAN'S INFLUENCE

My husband, Dr. Ryan Lazarus, is a functional medicine practitioner, nutrition expert, and motivational coach who is dedicated to redefining health through a holistic and transformative approach. His story is incredible; he survived a near-fatal sports accident at 18 that crushed his organs and has since lived with Type 1 diabetes and digestive failure, giving him a unique blend of professional expertise and personal resilience.

Ryan's personal journey fuels a deep passion for helping others unlock their full potential. Through optimal nutrition, strategic fitness programming, mental fitness techniques, strategic goal setting, and sustainable habit building, he empowers individuals to achieve lasting success in health, performance, and life transitions. I've leaned on him a lot and have always been inspired by his passion for helping and healing others.

A decade ago, he created The Lazarus Method, a holistic framework built on seven unique health elements designed for optimal health, performance, and life transformation. These seven health elements include Nourish, Rest, Move, Learn, Connect, Challenge and Spark and are all essential for holistic health and vitality.

In fact, we often discuss how my passion for setting inspiring running challenges encompasses all seven of these elements. While *movement* and training are fundamental, success also depends on proper *nutrition*, *rest*, and recovery. However, the less obvious elements may be the most crucial: *learning* from others and mentors, *connecting* to my inner voice, and leaning on my friends and family for support. The two most significant elements, *challenge* and *spark*, define my purpose for running and writing this book. Taking on massive challenges, fueled by my passion and the drive to reach my full potential, is what ignites my spark.

OFFENSE AND DEFENSE

Ryan suggests that life, much like a game, is a dynamic interplay between offense and defense. Offense is the proactive pursuit of progress, building momentum through structured routines, intentional health choices, and goal-driven actions. It's when you're in control, aligned with your priorities and purpose, and moving forward with confidence.

Defense, on the other hand, is the reactive side of life, where unpredictability forces adaptation. It's the moments of disruption—an illness, an injury, a work crisis, or personal struggles—that challenge your ability to stay on course. He believes the key to long-term success isn't avoiding defensive moments but recognizing that they are inevitable and preparing accordingly.

I had to put this concept to the test when, just one month before my 40th birthday run, I came down with the flu. It knocked me out for a week, and my immediate worry was that I had lost all the progress I had made in my training. But because I had been practicing both offense and defense, I was able to adapt. Instead of panicking, I shifted my focus to rest, hydration, and nutrition, trusting that recovery was just as important as the training itself. Letting go of the worry and fear was part of the process. At that moment, I was on defense, but I knew I'd soon be back on offense.

Momentum shifts between offense and defense are a universal experience, yet many, including both Ryan and I, can struggle when unexpectedly pushed into a reactive state. Without a solid game plan, people often abandon their goals and healthy habits and may fall back into unproductive patterns.

An effective health game plan is based on balance, flexibility, and consistency. This approach empowers you to sustain habits through any challenge, turn setbacks into resilience, and forge an unshakable foundation for lifelong vitality in health, performance, and life.

REASONS FOR CHANGE

According to leadership expert John Maxwell, people change when they:

- Hurt enough they have to
- See enough they are inspired to
- Learn enough that they want to
- Receive enough, they are able to

This framework can help you understand where *you* are in this process. Change is hard, but it is also inevitable.

GOING INWARD, THE ANTIDOTE

While leaning on support and turning to these frameworks are helpful, they're hard to do if we're constantly distracted. Going inward is the antidote. It's the practice of tuning out external chaos and reconnecting with our own thoughts, emotions, and intuition. It's not about escaping reality but rather about creating space to hear what truly matters. When we go inward, we find clarity, resilience, and a deep well of strength that no external validation can provide. It's in these still moments, whether through movement, breath, or solitude that we gain the awareness to navigate life with greater purpose and intention.

So, if you are able to quiet the noise, the next step is to gain clarity by going inward. There's no wrong way to do it, but if you need some guidance, see the following few examples.

RUNNING WITHOUT DISTRACTIONS

Instead of listening to music, a podcast, or tracking every mile, go for a run in silence. Feel your breath, the rhythm of your feet, and the way your body moves. This practice helps you tune into your own thoughts and emotions.

BREATHWORK AND MEDITATION

Start with 5 minutes of conscious breathing. Whether it's box breathing, alternate nostril breathing, or simply focusing on the inhale and exhale, this practice creates a direct connection between the mind and body, allowing for self-awareness and clarity.

SAUNA OR COLD PLUNGE REFLECTION

Instead of using your sauna or cold plunge as just a physical practice, treat it as a moment of mindfulness. In the heat, focus on releasing tension. In the cold, concentrate on steadying your breath and observing your thoughts without judgment.

JOURNALING AS A MIRROR

Write freely for five minutes without censoring yourself. Let your thoughts flow onto the page without worrying about structure or grammar. This is a way to see what's truly on your mind and heart.

TIME IN NATURE

Take a walk in nature alone without your phone. Observe the environment, feel your body moving through space, and let your thoughts settle. Being in nature naturally shifts you into a state of presence.

SITTING WITH DISCOMFORT

When facing a craving, an emotional trigger, or restlessness, instead of reaching for a distraction (food, social media, or an immediate fix), pause. Sit with it. Ask yourself, "What am I actually feeling?" Often, emotions reveal deeper needs when given space.

VISUALIZATION AND INTENTION-SETTING

Close your eyes and visualize yourself crossing a finish line, achieving a personal goal, or simply embodying your best self. This practice helps align your energy with your deeper purpose.

By focusing for just a few minutes every day on removing external distractions and reconnecting to your inner voice, you create space for intentionality, gain clarity, confidence, and the ability to pursue meaningful goals.

. . .

Pause & Reflect: What are the sources of "noise" in your life, such as social media, negative self-talk, or external pressures? What distractions keep you from your goal?

Coaching Advice: Commit to a mindfulness practice that helps you stay present and focused: meditation, breathwork, journaling or time in nature.

By clearing distractions, you create space for growth. Next, let's refine the tools in your toolbox to help you stay on track.

8

FIND YOUR ALIGNMENT

"Life is a balance between holding on and letting go."

RUMI

You already know my journey specific to running, and you may have noticed a theme of overtraining, under-fueling, and injury. For the first four decades of my life, I operated at one speed, the only one I knew: run fast, lift heavy, push hard, crash (get sick or injured), recover, rinse, and repeat. I was actually OK with this cycle because the crashes were minimal and infrequent. Usually, I was back at it in a few days. But coupled with the stress from my job, it just became too much, and it eventually caught up with me.

I tell this story because, looking back, I had only ever invested in certain "tools" in my "toolbox." My way of managing stress was to run, lift, hike, and get together with friends. It sounds like a good set of tools, right? Well, not if you are depleted and fatigued and your body can't physically manage the energy to do any of those activities.

It was time to find some new tools. Time to go inward. Time to rebalance.

Enter yoga.

I'm eternally grateful that in this time of rebalancing and discovery in my life, I found yoga. There were many mornings I would just show up on my mat and go through a minimal number of poses or sit with my thoughts and feel the small win of getting to class. I had always thought of yoga as boring and a waste of time; why would I do that when I could hit the trails and get my heart rate up? Looking back, it was what I had always needed to balance out my energy and make an investment in myself solely focused on rest, recovery, and restoration.

For months, yoga was my only form of activity. I just kept showing up on my mat, showing up for myself with a determination to heal my body, mind, and spirit and surrender to how long this may take. Seeing even small improvements in my overall wellbeing made me more curious about the history and philosophy of yoga. What's behind this powerful antidote that I had ignored for 42 years? I decided to go all in and enrolled in 200-hour yoga teacher training. I wanted to understand the meaning behind the poses, the healing properties of breathwork, and the thousand-year-old practice that had helped and healed so many.

THE WHEEL OF SUFFERING IN EVERYDAY LIFE

In my training, there were many concepts in yoga philosophy that spoke to me, but one in particular stood out: the Wheel of Suffering.

We all do it to ourselves in one way or another if we keep making the same choices or habits that lead to the same painful outcomes. It was one of those lessons I connected with immediately because, in hindsight, I could see where I was stuck. The Wheel of Suffering shows up for all of us in different ways; it's part of the human experience.

Ever feel like you're stuck in the same loop, repeating the same mistakes, habits, or emotional reactions, even when you know they don't serve you?

Perhaps you always start a new fitness routine but quit after two weeks. Or maybe you keep dating the same type of emotionally unavailable person, hoping "this time" will be different. Or you promise yourself you'll stop procrastinating but somehow always end up scrolling on your phone.

This is the Wheel of Suffering (Samsara) in action. It's not just a concept from yoga; it's the reality of unconscious patterns that keep us stuck in cycles of stress, frustration, and self-sabotage.

These cycles don't happen by accident; they're fueled by four common mental traps that keep us stuck.

1. We cling to comfort over growth, choosing what's familiar even when it holds us back.

2. We fear change because stepping into the unknown feels risky, even when we know staying the same isn't working.

3. Our ego identity convinces us that we're just "not that kind of person," whether it's waking up early, committing to

fitness, or building healthy relationships, so we reinforce old habits instead of shifting them.

4. When discomfort arises, we distract ourselves by procrastinating, scrolling, or numbing out instead of facing the real work.

The hard truth? Nothing changes unless we do.

Breaking free from the Wheel of Suffering starts with awareness. Once we start to recognize the toxic patterns that keep us stuck in cycles of stress, frustration, and self-sabotage, we can begin to break free from this cycle. Whether it's repeating unhealthy relationships, procrastinating on your goals, or numbing discomfort instead of facing it, these habits don't happen by accident. They're fueled by the need for comfort, fear of change, ego-driven identity, and avoidance of discomfort.

But awareness alone isn't enough; you need to build a toolbox of strategies to disrupt these patterns and create real change. Just as a runner trains with a variety of exercises to build strength, endurance and flexibility, you need different tools to tackle different challenges.

Mindfulness, movement, breathwork, self-reflection, and conscious habit shifts all act as tools to help you respond differently when old patterns try to pull you back in. The key is learning to reach for the right tool in the moment instead of falling back into automatic reactions. The more tools you build, the more resilient and adaptable you become, stepping off the hamster wheel of suffering and into a life of empowered action.

ADDING TOOLS TO YOUR TOOLBOX

Once I became aware of my ever-repeating cycle of push hard, crash (get sick or injured), recover, rinse, and repeat, I focused on adding more "tools" to my "toolbox." This list is taken directly from my journal during that time:

Previous tools: running, lifting, hiking, friends, family, healthy diet, gratitude

New tools: yoga, sauna, cold plunge, meditation, fasting, journaling, breathwork, evening walks, seeking information in the form of podcasts, books, and yoga philosophy to follow my curiosity, an open mind, and surrender.

The realization came in the form of balance. Everything in nature craves balance, and our bodies and minds are no different. I had been on a path that was moving at such a fast speed that I didn't take the necessary time to slow down, rest, recover, and go inward.

INHALE THE GOOD SHIT, EXHALE THE BULLSHIT

If you can add one thing to your toolbox, let it be breathwork. While we might not all have access to sauna and cold plunge, we all have access to our breath. It costs nothing and takes only a few seconds to make a huge impact. There are many breathwork techniques designed to either energize you or help you relax. Breathwork is a powerful tool to anchor you in the present moment, and one of the simplest ways to begin is by taking just three deep breaths.

THE IMPORTANCE OF
MOVEMENT DIVERSITY

This personal experience of overtraining and crashing is why, as a coach, I emphasize the diversity of movement and the importance of mindfulness for long-term physical and mental health. Balance is the harmonious integration of physical, mental, and emotional health, and your workouts should properly support all three of these aspects. Here's why:

- **Avoiding Plateaus:** By varying your activities, you can help prevent injury and burnout and instead promote growth in varied muscle groups and skills. It will also allow you to pivot as challenges come up, like injury, illness, or travel.

- **Cross-Training Benefits:** Incorporating strength, endurance, flexibility and mindfulness into your routine leads to balanced training for holistic fitness. Think of it this way: the goal is to have the energy to chase after your kids or grandkids, lift them into their car seats, and have the mindfulness to transform their screaming in the car into a moment of presence and gratitude.

- **Mental Fitness:** Learning new physical skills (dance, yoga, martial arts, etc.) enhances brain health and mental agility. Building a new skill takes effort, forces us to step outside our comfort zone, and can also lead to a new hobby and social network.

- **Breaking Monotony:** Diversity of activities keeps workouts engaging and sustainable. The goal is to be able to "workout" and enjoy movement for the rest of your life. The only way to do this is to keep it fresh, incorporate new skills and keep your body and mind engaged and healthy along the way. If you're not having fun, rethink your movement patterns. It should be equally challenging and enjoyable if you want to build something sustainable.

BALANCE IN THE BODY:

Strength and Flexibility: Think of the opposites as a pair for balance. On your strength days, you build stability, and by adding flexibility, you can lessen stiffness and avoid injury. Combine your heavy lifting or strength workouts with foam rolling, stretching or yoga, targeting the same muscle groups you've just challenged in your workout.

Endurance and Recovery: Cardio is essential for health and can be incredibly beneficial across all five heart rate zones. In the lower heart rate zones (1–3), you go low and slow for longer periods of time. In the higher zones (4–5), you hit that heart rate threshold, recruiting from the anaerobic energy system. In both scenarios, you need the balance of rest or "active recovery" to promote muscle repair and maintain mental clarity to avoid burnout.

Core Stability: We need our core for everything! The core is the foundation for all movement, linking our upper and lower body strength and preventing injury to the lower back and spine. Incorporate planks, stability ball exercises and good old-fashioned sit-ups into your routine to maintain a healthy and strong core.

BALANCE IN THE MIND:

Mind-Body Connection: It's sometimes easy to disconnect the two, thinking of your day in sections. First, I'll go to the gym and work on my body; then, I'll transition to work and use my mind. However, they are, in fact, always connected and more powerful when they are continuously communicating with each other. Practices like yoga, Tai Chi and breathwork help build that connection, improve focus, and reduce overall stress.

Mental Flexibility: Engaging in new physical challenges also challenges the agility of our mind and can strengthen cognitive resilience. Think back to the chapter on goal setting; if you've practiced mental fitness by learning new sports or skills, you will be more open to trying a new challenge or setting a ceiling goal, because you won't be as afraid to fail.

Mental Clarity: We've talked about rest and recovery in the form of movement, but sometimes, the best way to rest is not moving at all. Sleep is essential for repair and recovery, and the lack of it can lead to injury and illness. In addition to a good night's sleep, meditation, mindfulness, and breathwork are great tools to create a balanced and healthy mental state.

STEPS TO ACHIEVE BALANCE:

Create a Movement Menu: Write out five different activities you enjoy, like walking, hiking with friends, swimming, strength training, yoga, or just playing outside. Make an effort to incorporate and vary each activity throughout the week. Make sure you check in with yourself daily and pivot if you need a yoga day instead of a 10-mile run; you now have more tools in your toolbox, so make sure you reach for the one that's the best fit for that day.

Schedule Active Recovery Days: Write out five restorative activities that you enjoy. Here's a tip: if you can only think of one or two, it's time to focus on that mental fitness piece and learn some new skills. Here are a few ideas to get you started: walking in nature, stretching, Tai Chi, yoga, foam rolling, walking meditation or an easy hike with friends.

Mindful Integration: Practice mindfulness during your physical activity to align your body and mind. This requires an honest check-in with yourself: Is this activity moving you closer to achieving your goal? Do you feel aligned with your compass? Are you celebrating your successes as you meet your floor goals? Are you showing up for these activities in balance with your intrinsic and extrinsic motivators?

Give yourself grace in this process; it may take some experimentation to find what works for you. Sara's story is an example of how a personal restorative practice can create presence of body and mind.

BENDING WITHOUT BREAKING: SARA'S STORY

I step onto my mat, feeling the tightness in my body before I even begin. But today, I'm not just here to stretch my muscles; I'm here to stretch my mind.

Lately, life has felt rigid: too many things on the "to-do" list, not enough time in the day. Every unexpected turn, every challenge, has made me feel like I might snap under the pressure. But today, I have a different intention. I want to become more flexible, not just in my body, but in my mindset.

I start in a simple forward fold, but my hamstrings protest immediately. I resist, gripping my muscles as if control will make this easier. I hear the instructor say, "Inhale, and as you exhale, deepen into the stretch." This is hard. Isn't this what I do in life, too? Cling too tightly instead of letting things unfold? I exhale and release, sinking deeper. The moment I stop fighting, space opens up.

Each pose is this way: I can feel the tension from my spine, the resistance in my muscles. The instructor encourages, "Inhale, and as you exhale, let go of anything that doesn't serve you." Breathe and let go, I tell myself. Each breath out carries away the frustration, the need to control, the old patterns that no longer serve me.

By the time I reach Savasana, my body feels lighter, but more importantly, so does my mind. I spent the last hour training my body and my mind to surrender and to be present. My "to-do" list flashes back in my mind, but it doesn't carry the same weight that it did just an hour before.

THE GIFT OF BALANCE

The benefit of balance and diversity in your movement is like writing a check to your future self. Some of this investment you won't be able to see or feel for years to come, but trust that there is no better gift to yourself than a balanced body, mind, and spirit.

Incorporating movement diversity and balance into your routine will translate into greater adaptability and resilience in life, and this is crucial as we all move through different life stages that require us to level up in new and demanding ways.

• • •

Pause & Reflect: Are there areas of your life that feel unbalanced? Are you repeating any patterns that don't serve you?

Coaching Advice: Make a list of all the tools and habits you currently rely on. Now, add three new ones that will help you break free from old cycles. These could include:

1. A new accountability partner

2. A habit-tracking system

3. A mindfulness or self-care practice

Now that you've built a stronger foundation, let's zoom out and reflect on the bigger picture.

9

TRUST YOUR POWER

*"Twenty years from now, you will be more disappointed
by the things you didn't do than by the ones you did."*

MARK TWAIN

There comes a moment in every transformational journey where
you have to take a leap of faith. For me, that moment was sign-
ing up for The Great World Race, a commitment that would challenge everything I thought I was capable of.

By now, you've gotten to know the real me, someone who's been on
a journey of identity and self-discovery, reclaiming my health and
searching for purpose in my current stage of life. Part of this process
for me was to take a GIANT leap of faith, one that would force me
to clean out and clean up all the distractions in my life and put me
on a path that would require me to be 100% focused and determined
in pursuit of my dream. I would have to face all my fears, overcome
self-doubt, and make big changes in my career in order to chase this
dream. In December of 2024, the week before Christmas, I signed

up for The Great World Race, and for the first time in a long time, I bet on myself.

The Great World Race is seven marathons in seven days on seven continents. It's important to go back to the beginning, remember my mostly average running journey, and distinguish that I am in no way a professional athlete. This race is my dream. I can't quite put into words why I chose this race specifically, but as soon as I learned about it the year before, I just couldn't get it out of my mind. It was equally exciting and terrifying, and that is a good barometer if you're looking for a life-transforming challenge.

When I first learned about this race, it seemed like there were only obstacles in the way. It was a very costly event, and we didn't have the extra funds in our savings. Additionally, it would demand a level of mental and physical commitment that felt akin to taking on another full-time job, and I simply didn't have the time for that. Also, why did I even think this was possible? At this point, I'd only run one marathon horribly, and I'd had a history of overtraining and injury. But something deep inside me knew this was my path and my journey to share. If I can dream this dream and have the confidence to chase it, maybe someone else will be inspired to chase theirs.

Fear of failure, imposter syndrome, and financial or logistical barriers often hold people back from taking bold action. I know firsthand how easy it is to second-guess yourself when stepping into the unknown, when the path ahead is uncertain, and there's no guarantee of success. The mind clings to comfort, preferring the familiarity of struggle over the risk of change. Doubts whisper, "What if I'm not good enough? What if I fail? What if I lose everything?"

These fears threatened to keep me stuck, convincing me that playing it safe is better than facing potential disappointment. But for me, and for many, real failure isn't about falling short; it's about never trying at all. Growth demands a leap of faith, a willingness to embrace discomfort, and the courage to bet on yourself, even when no one else does. The truth is, success isn't about having a perfect plan or eliminating fear; it's about moving forward despite it.

WHAT IS YOUR INNER RACE?

Setting an inspiring movement goal is so powerful that it will inevitably create positive change on the inside as well as the outside. Now that you've been working with your inspiring movement goal, I want you to take inventory and see if any larger desires or dreams are surfacing because that's how this process works. The inner spark is contagious, and it keeps revealing more of your truth. Take inventory of any larger fears that are holding you back from becoming the person you're meant to be. What dreams and longings are you ready to name? What fears, doubts, or self-imposed limits are you ready to confront?

The Inner Race is about uncovering what truly excites you, what aligns with your values, and what brings you closer to your authentic self. While the external victories will be celebrated along the way, only you will know the true prize: the unshakeable confidence and peace that comes from running your race, your way, and crossing a finish line only you can see.

POWER OF PERSONAL GROWTH

There is an entire industry focused on selling us "personal growth" advice. You could choose from countless books or spend hours listening to podcasts that offer similar advice, presented in various ways, and they are not wrong. The reason there is a huge market for personal growth advice is because there is a huge need for it. We all strive to become the best versions of ourselves and to move from challenging situations to awareness and growth.

The best way to harness your own power of personal growth is not necessarily through someone else's advice (mine included). You already have all the answers you're looking for within you. However, this next part takes work; it's not as simple as just pressing play on a podcast.

YOUR INNER GUIDE

Only you know the best way to go inward and connect with your intuition and inner guidance, also known as the little voice inside. There are an endless number of ways to go inward, such as journaling, meditation, listening to music, embracing stillness, or seeking solitude. Just find the one that speaks to you.

When I first began this journey, these were all very hard for me. I was out of practice and used to a pace of life that didn't allow for quiet moments of reflection. I was especially frustrated when trying to meditate. After just a few moments, a part of me would become frustrated and judgmental. I wanted to master this skill and control the experience. I kept asking myself, "Why can't I quiet my thoughts? Am I sitting the right way? Shouldn't I be feeling something by now? Why am I not having an amazing spiritual experience?" I had this overwhelming feeling that I was "doing it wrong." And I quit many times.

This was until I had a casual conversation with a new friend, Jon, who happens to be a meditation expert. He was practicing Tai Chi on the beach, and I had just finished a run. As we began our walk back to meet the group, he asked me about life, and I explained that I had always wanted to learn how to meditate, but I just couldn't grasp it. It seemed like it should be so easy, and I conceptually understood the life-changing benefits. He listened with patience and offered me the simplest advice: "There is no perfect way to meditate. Just start and start small. Meditate for one second." This was a lightbulb moment for me. It took the pressure off and allowed me to try again with this new "floor" goal and let go of judgment.

Since then, I've often leaned on the practice of meditation, especially in moments when doubt arises, or I'm seeking clarity and guidance. Some mornings, I have thirty minutes to devote to it; other times, it's just a brief moment of presence and awareness. As I prepare for the physical, mental, and emotional journey of The Great World Race, I know this practice will be a vital tool to help me adapt to the challenges that will arise during training and the race itself.

INTRINSIC MOTIVATION AND EXTERNAL EXPECTATIONS

Internal motivators are incredibly powerful when making big life decisions. The sense of achievement that comes from overcoming obstacles, like that "I did it" feeling, serves as a strong validation of alignment and purpose. This sense of fulfillment is the foundation necessary to chase that big dream with confidence. On the flip side, it's also important to navigate the external expectations, opinions, and pressures.

You can imagine that even though I was clear this race was my dream and "rite of passage" into this next stage of my life, it was met with a lot of skepticism from people in my inner circle. I was very careful to hold on tight to this dream and quietly do the inner work for months before sharing it with anyone. I needed to work through my own doubts, fears, and reasons for doing this race. Just like my 40th birthday run, I was afraid if I shared it too early, I'd let my own self-doubt get in the way and move on to an easier, more achievable goal. Fear of failure is real, and our ego protects us from scary situations that eventually lead to growth and some of the most incredible journeys in life.

IMPOSTER SYNDROME

Imposter syndrome, when it comes to chasing your dreams, is the persistent feeling that you're not truly capable or deserving of the success you're pursuing, despite clear evidence to the contrary. It's the voice in your head that whispers, "Who do you think you are to do this? You're not qualified enough, talented enough, or experienced enough." For me, it usually creeps in around 2 a.m., when the house is quiet and dark, and the only voice I hear is in my head.

It shows up when you take a risk, step outside your comfort zone, or go after something bigger than you've done before. Instead of feeling excited, you feel like a fraud, like at any moment, someone will "find out" that you don't belong.

But here's the truth: Imposter syndrome doesn't mean you're not capable. It means you're growing. It means you care. It means you're stepping into something that challenges you.

The key isn't to eliminate imposter syndrome when those doubts creep in; it's to keep going anyway. The people who achieve their dreams aren't necessarily the ones who never doubt themselves; they're the ones who feel the doubt and still take the next step.

Committing to running The Great World Race required me to push past self-doubt, navigate skepticism from others, and fully trust in my ability to follow through. It reinforced the power of betting on yourself, even when the outcome is uncertain.

"When the why is clear, the how becomes eas(ier)"

JIM ROHN

I had sat with this dream long enough; I was clear on my why. Now, it was time to put it into motion. First, I told my husband, "I'm going to run this race; it's seven marathons in seven days on seven continents." His reaction was pretty normal and unsurprising; he rolled his eyes and dismissed the idea, thinking I was totally nuts. However, when he understood my "why," he became my number one supporter. Then I told my kids, my parents, my sister, and my running friends. I was almost pressure-testing the idea, trying to gauge reactions. How would these people who know me best react? If they didn't believe in me, could I still believe in myself?

It's very common to fear judgment, even when we are the most confident version of ourselves. This was something I had let get in my way for too long. In order to move forward and release this need for approval and fear of falling short of expectations, I had to accept that failure (not completing the race) was a possibility. I realized that the real failure would be not chasing after my dream, not seeking my full potential, not prioritizing my own growth, and not teaching my kids that anything is possible.

So, I laid down all my chips, financially, emotionally, and physically, and I bet on myself.

BETTING ON YOURSELF

There's a reason why I decided to write this book while training for The Great World Race instead of after finishing the race. I believe the best lessons are learned from the journey. The risk, courage, and focus that's cultivated just by making a decision to go after your goal is the true gift. I can feel the power of this gift taking shape in my own life, and the race is still months away. Wherever you are in life and whatever goal you've set for yourself, have faith that the transformation is already underway.

Make that bet on yourself! In the past few chapters, you've clarified your goals, reflected on your current stage in life, and thought about your "why." The next step is to act on this goal and commit to writing the next chapter of your life's story. Let's pause for a moment for a meditation exercise; this is a very helpful and well-known meditation that will help you reflect on the chapters of your life, connect to the place you are at, and clarify where you want to go next.

THE BOOK OF LIFE MEDITATION EXERCISE

The "Book of Life" meditation is most commonly associated with Michael Singer, the author of *The Untethered Soul*. In his teachings, he describes a meditation practice where you view your life as if it were a book, turning the pages without attachment, allowing each moment to pass without resistance.

Let's begin:

- Sit comfortably and take a deep breath. Imagine you are holding a large, beautifully bound book, the book of your life.

- Gently open it to the first pages. See the memories of your childhood, the people who shaped you, the moments of laughter and innocence. Flip through the chapters of your youth, your struggles, your victories, the lessons you've learned.

- Now, arrive at the present moment, the page you are on today. Feel the weight of your journey, the wisdom you carry, and the possibilities ahead.

- Turn to the next page. It is blank and waiting to be written. What will you create? Who will you become? What dreams will you chase?

- Take a deep breath and visualize yourself writing the next chapter with intention, courage, and inspiration.

- When you're ready, gently close the book, knowing that your story is still unfolding and you are the author.

Take one more deep breath. Take note of how you feel after this exercise.

Carry this awareness with you, and step forward into the next page of your life.

• • •

Pause & Reflect: In the "Book of Life" exercise, how did it feel to reflect on your journey? What emotions surfaced when you realized there are still unwritten chapters?

Coaching Advice: It's time to quiet external noise, fears, doubts, and limiting beliefs and fully commit to your goal.

1. Revisit your goal. Does it align with your core values?

2. Develop a daily reflection habit using affirmations, meditation, or gratitude journaling.

3. Take one bold action today that moves your goal forward.

Your goal is no longer just an idea; it's something you are actively working toward! Now, let's celebrate your progress and take action on your new challenge in the final chapters.

10

FINISH STRONG

"The top of one mountain is the
bottom of the next, so keep climbing."

ANDRÉ DE SHIELDS

THE FINISH LINE IS ONLY THE BEGINNING

For years, I searched desperately for my "purpose." The word felt so daunting, and I feared making the wrong choice. What if my purpose wasn't grand enough? What if it changed? What if I failed? Then, I came across a message in the book *Travel Light* by Light Watkins, the author and meditation expert, who shifted everything for me. His message is, "Follow your curiosity." At that moment, just like the simple meditation advice from my friend Jon, the heavy burden I had placed on myself lifted, and the search for purpose became much simpler and more exciting.

I started small. I was curious about fitness, so I got certified. I was curious about coaching and excited to share what I'd learned, so I started teaching classes. I was drawn to yoga, so I studied its philosophy and began applying it to my life. I followed my curiosity wherever it led me without forcing any grand vision. It wasn't about having all the answers. It was about trusting the process and letting life unfold as I kept following what lit me up. Today, my curiosity drives me to explore what happens when I take risks, remove mental barriers, and empower others to do the same.

YOUR OWN JOURNEY

I want to encourage you to apply this same mindset to your own journey, whether you are just beginning or have been on the path of exploring deeper meaning for a long time. Too often, we think of success as a destination, some final "finish line" that, once crossed, will bring all the answers. But what if we reframe it? The finish line is not the end; it's just another beginning. Every step you take toward your goal is a step toward deeper understanding, growth, and fulfillment. Your journey will be dynamic, and your purpose may evolve as you move forward. And that's okay. The important thing is to stay curious, stay open, and trust that the right steps will reveal themselves as you continue to move forward.

You've taken time to reflect on what naturally inspires you, what lights you up. These sparks of curiosity, no matter how small, hold the key to unlocking your unique path forward and can guide you along the way. Remember, your journey doesn't have to be perfect, and it doesn't follow any timeline. *The process is where the magic happens.*

As discussed in the previous chapter, you may also encounter fear and self-doubt along the way. These emotions are a natural part of the journey and don't mean you're on the wrong path. Instead of trying to avoid them, lean into them. Fear is simply a sign that you're pushing the boundaries of your comfort zone, which is exactly where growth happens. Don't let it stop you from moving forward. Keep taking small steps. Celebrate your wins, no matter how small they seem, and acknowledge that each moment brings you closer to your true potential.

THE RIPPLE EFFECT

Remember that any and all progress you make on your very personal journey is worth celebrating. By taking action and following your inspiration, you may also notice the ripple effect in those around you. This is magic! As you begin your journey, harness your power, and start making strides, others will take notice, and you never know who you may inspire along the way.

Erika's story is an example of this ripple effect in action. She was ready to make improvements in her own life and even knew how to do it; she just needed a little nudge of inspiration.

STEPS TO SUCCESS: ERIKA'S STORY

Erika, a friend and coworker, had never been one for fitness challenges. She had tried countless times to stick to a workout routine, but nothing ever worked. Life always got in the way.

Like many busy working moms, it felt like there were always more urgent things to handle: emails to answer, lunches to pack, and kids to shuttle from one activity to the next. Exercise always got pushed to the bottom of the "to-do" list.

So, when she heard about my training for The Great World Race, she was intrigued and excited for me. The logistical feat of the race sounded impossible. But as we talked about my reason for choosing this challenge, and how goal setting wasn't just about the achievement but about the transformation along the way, something clicked for her. A few days later, she sent me a text.

"I'm not running marathons, but I can walk 10,000 steps. I'm starting today."

For Erika, this was huge. She implemented small changes like taking her dog for an extra walk, parking further away at the grocery store, squeezing in walks between conference calls. She started noticing how much better she felt after each walk. The stress of the day didn't weigh as heavily, and she actually looked forward to the time outside, just for herself.

Weeks later, she told me, "I never thought I'd be the kind of person who actually sticks to a goal like this. But here I am."

She wasn't just walking; she was proving to herself that she could commit to something, that her health did matter, and that real change starts with one small step.

It's incredibly powerful and humbling to know that, in some small way, my taking action on my goal has inspired her to do the same. We all have the ability to inspire and empower others through our actions, and you never know who may need that bit of encouragement as your ripple effect begins.

THE POWER IS IN THE JOURNEY

As much as I love running, it's not about crossing a single finish line. There's always another race, another goal on the horizon. In the same way, life is a continuous journey of growth, discovery, and reinvention. There will always be another "finish line" to cross, but the true rewards come from the process itself: the learning, the perseverance, and the moments where you break through your own limits.

When you run, you don't just focus on reaching the finish line; you focus on how you run, the rhythm of your breath, the steadiness of your pace, and the strength in each step. The journey is where you truly find your power, not just in the end result. Similarly, in life, it's not solely about reaching a particular goal or defining success in a single moment. It's about how you show up along the way, how you learn to navigate obstacles, and how you keep pushing yourself forward even when it feels hard. Every step matters, and each step shapes who you become.

The finish line is just a checkpoint, a moment to pause, reflect, and then begin again. Life is the same. Once you cross one finish line, you find another one waiting for you. But it's the journey between those lines that truly matters. The beauty of life lies in our ability to evolve, adjust our pace, and challenge ourselves with new goals. So, remember that the finish line is not an endpoint; it's an opportunity to begin again, stronger, wiser, and better prepared for whatever comes next.

• • •

Pause & Reflect: Looking back on your journey, what accomplishment are you most proud of? How will you celebrate your progress while setting your sights on the next challenge?

Coaching Advice: The finish line is just another milestone, not the end.

1. Reflect: Are you ready to begin your movement challenge?

2. Celebrate: Acknowledge your growth. Setting your inspired challenge is a milestone!

3. Empower: Share your success with a friend! You can be the inspiration for someone else to begin their own journey.

This is just the beginning. Keep chasing challenges that inspire you, keep moving, and keep redefining what's possible in the pursuit of running your own inner race.

11

OWN YOUR RACE

*"Do not go where the path may lead, go instead
where there is no path and leave a trail."*

RALPH WALDO EMERSON

t's 6 a.m. on a Sunday morning. The sky is still dark, and the world feels quiet, except in downtown Oakland, where the marathon start line is alive with energy. There is a combination of nervous anticipation and excitement as thousands of runners gather, each with their own personal goal. Some have trained diligently through the cold winter months, driven by the pursuit of a personal record. Others are here to conquer the full 26.2 miles for the very first time, a challenge that represents more than just distance, but also dedication, hard work, and growth.

Despite our diverse backgrounds and reasons for being here, we all share a common purpose that unites us. Each of us understands, in our own way, what it took to arrive at this moment: the early mornings, sore muscles, moments of doubt, and quiet perseverance. As we stand together in the early morning chill, we are collectively aware that the hours ahead will test us. Yet, we've shown up, ready to rise to the challenge.

For me, this marathon is a chance to shake off the dust of a failed marathon attempt nearly two decades ago. My intention is to use the Oakland Marathon as a training milestone for The Great World Race. I plan to run it slowly, finish strong, and build the confidence I'll need to complete seven consecutive marathons this coming November.

I have no idea what the next 26.2 miles will hold, but I already know this journey has changed me in ways I never could have imagined.

And just before the starting gun goes off and I'm put to the test, I pause for a moment of gratitude for the process, the growth, and the path that brought me here. Because, in many ways, I already feel like I've won.

• • •

The Inner Race is not measured by miles, medals, or records; it's the unseen journey that takes place within. It's the journey that challenges us to confront our fears, push through self-imposed limits, and find more clarity and alignment in life.

It is a race of purpose, not performance.

This journey is deeply personal, fueled by internal motivation rather than external rewards. It's about showing up for yourself when no one is watching, staying committed through challenges, and discovering meaning in the process rather than the outcome.

In the *Inner Race*, the journey itself is the reward. In the moments of discomfort, you uncover your resilience. It's the small, consistent wins—the early mornings, the extra steps, and the decision to believe in yourself, even when it feels impossible—that reveal the true victory: your personal growth.

In this book, you've taken time to reflect on what brings you joy in this stage of life, identified the barriers that hold you back, and developed tools to help you navigate challenges as they arise.

Now, it's time to take the next step. You've chosen your inspiring movement challenge and are ready to ignite your inner spark!

By taking even the smallest step toward change, you've invested in yourself. Life will always present challenges, doubts, and fears, but those obstacles are what make the journey meaningful. You have everything you need within you to cross any finish line and begin new chapters with confidence.

The goal isn't simply to reach the end of the race; it's to live fully and authentically along the way.

As you move forward, remember that the finish line is only the beginning. Life is a series of steps, each one leading you toward your next adventure. Embrace the path ahead. Follow your curiosity. Let your momentum grow.

You are capable of far more than you know. The world is waiting for you to light that spark within and share your unique gifts. The more you follow your heart, the clearer your path will become.

As we come to the end of this book, I want to leave you with a final thought, one that reflects the essence of *The Inner Race*, and the words I use to close every yoga class:

> **May your thoughts inspire you.**
>
> **May your words empower you.**
>
> **May your heart guide you.**

Chase your new goal with courage, and shine your light brightly, because when you do, you give others permission to find and shine theirs too.

ABOUT THE AUTHOR

Natalia is married to Ryan and is the proud mother of two teenagers, Cienna and Easton, three if you count her golden retriever, Charlie. She is a health coach for The Lazarus Method, a local fitness instructor, an ultra-distance runner, and a dedicated yogi.

Natalia's journey in health and fitness is deeply integrated with her love for nature and adventure. Some of her favorite activities include family travels to National Parks in their Sprinter van, hiking trips with her friends, and exploring new places around the world, all of which fuel her holistic approach to health. Her philosophy is rooted in the belief that life is an adventure and that we all deserve to chase our dreams.

Natalia is currently training for The Great World Race, a once-in-a-lifetime event that combines her passion for running and travel. The race consists of seven marathons in seven days on all seven continents.

www.ingramcontent.com/pod-product-compliance
Lightning Source LLC
Chambersburg PA
CBHW032041040426
42449CB00007B/973